W9-BKF-620

Contents

Student Study Guide

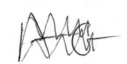

FUNDAMENTALS OF NURSING

STANDARDS & PRACTICE

SECOND EDITION

Sue C. DeLaune, MN, RN, C
Adjunct Faculty
Loyola University
New Orleans, Louisiana
President, SDeLaune Consulting
Mandeville, Louisiana
Health Education Coordinator
Southeast Louisiana Hospital
Mandeville, Louisiana

Patricia K. Ladner, MS, MN, RN
Consultant for Nursing Practice
Louisiana State Board of Nursing
New Orleans, Louisiana

Questions Prepared by

Marilyn Stapleton, MS, RN, C
Nurse Educator, Excelsior College School of Nursing
Albany, NY

DELMAR
™
THOMSON LEARNING

Australia Canada Mexico Singapore Spain United Kingdom United States

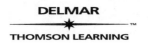

DELMAR
THOMSON LEARNING

Student Study Guide
Fundamentals of Nursing: Standards and Practice
Second Edition

by Sue C. DeLaune and Patricia K. Ladner
Questions prepared by Marilyn Stapleton

Health Care Publishing Director:
William Brottmiller

Executive Editor:
Cathy L. Esperti

Acquisitions Editor:
Matthew Filimonov

Developmental Editor:
Patricia A. Gaworecki

Editorial Assistant:
Melissa Longo

Executive Marketing Manager:
Dawn F. Gerrain

Channel Manager:
Jennifer McAvey

Project Editor:
Mary Ellen Cox

Production Editor:
James Zayicek

Art/Design Coordinator:
Connie Lundberg-Watkins

For permission to use material from this text or product, contact us by
Tel   (800) 730-2214
Fax   (800) 730-2215
www.thomsonrights.com

ISBN: 0-7668-2453-5

NOTICE TO THE READER

Publisher does not warrant or guarantee any of the products described herein or perform any independent analysis in connection with any of the product information contained herein. Publisher does not assume, and expressly disclaims, any obligation to obtain and include information other than that provided to it by the manufacturer.

The reader is expressly warned to consider and adopt all safety precautions that might be indicated by the activities herein and to avoid all potential hazards. By following the instructions contained herein, the reader willingly assumes all risks in connection with such instructions.

The Publisher makes no representation or warranties of any kind, including but not limited to, the warranties of fitness for particular purpose or merchantability, nor are any such representations implied with respect to the material set forth herein, and the publisher takes no responsibility with respect to such material. The publisher shall not be liable for any special, consequential, or exemplary damages resulting, in whole or part, from the readers' use of, or reliance upon, this material.

Chapter 1   Evolution of Nursing and Health Care

1. Nurses focus on a client's

   a. illness.

   b. response to illness.

2. In the early 1800s, nursing was primarily work performed in the home by female caretakers.

   ❑ True

   ❑ False

3. There is evidence that suggests women, as nurses, were empowered by their religious affiliation to provide health care services during the 1800s and 1900s.

   ❑ True

   ❑ False

4. Florence Nightingale revolutionized nursing by

   a. establishing the first hospital in Britain where nurses could practice without the direction of physicians.

   b. changing the image of nurses from handmaidens to professionals with autonomy.

   c. educating nurses in theoretical concepts as well as clinical skills.

   d. developing the first documentation system for patient care.

5. Which of the following women in nursing history founded the Red Cross in the United States?

   a. Dorothea Dix

   b. Lillian Wald

   c. Annie Goodrich

   d. Clara Barton

6. Which of the following nursing leaders founded several nursing organizations and supported the rights of nursing students?

    a. Isabell Hampton Robb

    b. Adelaide Nutting

    c. Jane Delano

    d. Lavinia Dock

7. The American Nurses Association (ANA) was founded in 1903.

    ❏ True

    ❏ False

8. Match the decade in the left column with the event that occurred in that decade from the right column.

_____ 1920s	a.	Proliferation of HMOs
_____ 1930s	b.	Creation of Medicare and Medicaid
_____ 1940s	c.	The Brown Report
_____ 1950s	d.	Women can vote
_____ 1960s	e.	The advent of Blue Cross and Blue Shield
_____ 1970s	f.	The advent of LPN programs
_____ 1980s	g.	Health care reform
_____ 1990s	h.	Nurse practitioners reimbursed directly for their services

9. Which of the following nursing leaders established the Frontier Nursing Service, thereby introducing health care delivery to rural America?

    a. Mary Breckinridge

    b. Adelaide Nutting

    c. Clara Barton

    d. Lavinia Dock

10. Margaret Sanger is known for her activist work around the issue of birth control in the early 1900s.

    ❏ True

    ❏ False

11. There were several landmark reports about medical and nursing education that brought about changes in nursing. Match the report with its focus listed in the right column.

_____	Flexner Report	a.	Identified a shortage of nurses in teaching, research, and administration
_____	Goldmark Report	b.	Brought accountability to medical education
_____	Brown Report	c.	Identified the need for greater professional competence in nursing, recommended moving nursing education from hospitals to the university setting
_____	Nursing and Nursing Education: Public Policies and Private Actions	d.	Identified major weaknesses in the hospital-based nursing programs

12. Which of the following nursing pioneers suggested the establishment of a national health insurance plan?

a. Isabel Hampton Robb

b. Lillian Wald

c. Adelaide Nutting

d. Mary Mahoney

13. The main reason for the growth of insurance plans in the 1920s was

a. physician advocacy.

b. the influence of Metropolitan Insurance Company.

c. the Depression.

d. pressure from hospitals.

14. The proliferation of Practical Nursing Programs was spurred by the need for health care providers who would work at a lower wage than RNs.

❑ True

❑ False

15. Nursing's early link with religious organizations had a negative impact on the development of nursing as a profession.

❑ True

❑ False

16. The Joint Commission on the Accreditation of Healthcare Organizations (JACHO) plays a direct role in the improvement of the quality of health care delivery in the U.S. by viewing quality as

    a. an outcome.

    b. procedure oriented.

    c. person centered.

    d. related to the ratio of uninsured to insured Americans.

17. The major goals of Healthy People 2010 are to increase quality and years of healthy life and to eliminate health disparities.

    ❏ True

    ❏ False

18. The future of nursing will benefit from differentiated practice models as new graduates enter the employment arena.

    ❏ True

    ❏ False

19. Considering the evolution of nursing as a profession, is there a relationship between the empowerment of nurses and the autonomy nurses feel individually and collectively?

    ❏ Yes

    ❏ No

20. Evidence-based nursing practice can be best described as

    a. collecting data to support medical practice.

    b. clinical decision making by nurse scholars based on empirical evidence.

    c. the joint development of nursing and medical science.

    d. the application of evidence from research findings to aid in clinical decision making.

Chapter 2   Theoretical Foundations of Nursing

1. Match the definitions from the right column with the terms in the left column.

    _____ concept   a. The use of formalized methods to generate information about a phenomenon

    _____ phenomenon   b. A relational statement that links concepts

    _____ proposition   c. Basic building block of theory

    _____ theory   d. Field of study

    _____ discipline   e. An observable fact that can be perceived through the senses and explained

    _____ research   f. Describes, explains, or predicts situations

2. Nursing practice, theory, and research exist

    a. independently of each other.

    b. as a closely related whole.

    c. in a loosely linked relationship.

3. Which of the following would represent a grand nursing theory?

    a. Peplau's Theory of Interpersonal Relations

    b. Orem's Self-Care Deficit Theory of Nursing

    c. Nightingale's Notes on Nursing

    d. Abdellah's 21 Nursing Problems

4. Nursing theory development and research activities are directed toward

    _____.

5. The unifying force in a discipline that names the phenomena of concern to that discipline is called a

    a. paradigm.

    b. metaparadigm.

    c. framework.

    d. model.

6. Middle-range nursing theory can be derived from a grand nursing theory.

   ❑ True

   ❑ False

7. According to Fawcett, the major concepts that provide structure to the domain of nursing are

   a. patient, environment, health, nursing.

   b. nursing, client, environment, health.

   c. person, environment, nursing, well-being.

   d. person, environment, health, nursing.

8. According to Parse, there are two paradigms in nursing. The paradigm that defines the person as "more than the sum of the parts and is constantly changing . . . co-creating health through mutual interchange with the environment" is the

   a. Simultaneity Paradigm.

   b. Totality Paradigm.

9. Which of the following nursing theorists put forward the following definition of nursing? "The unique function of the nurse is to assist the individual, sick or well, in the performance of those activities contributing to health or its recovery (or to peaceful death) that he would perform unaided if he had the necessary strength, will, or knowledge."

   a. Florence Nightingale

   b. Jean Watson

   c. Myra Levine

   d. Virginia Henderson

10. Mr. O'Grady is recovering from an aortic aneurysm repair. His recovery is complicated by a residual difficulty to swallow, possibly secondary to a minor CVA during surgery. The speech therapist has placed him on a swallowing protocol, whereby he is relearning how to swallow. As a nurse, you are supporting this adaptive behavior, which fosters optimal functioning. Which of the following theories would best describe the theoretical framework you will be operating through as you support his coping?

    a. Orem's Self-Care Deficit Theory of Nursing

    b. The Roy Adaptation Model

    c. Watson's Theory of Human Caring

11. Nursing theory exists without the need for validity testing through nursing research.

    ❑ True

    ❑ False

12. Which of the following nursing theorists is concerned with a humanistic-altruistic philosophical basis for the science of nursing as well as the classification of caring behaviors?

    a. Jean Watson

    b. Martha Rogers

    c. Rosemarie Parse

    d. Dorothea Orem

13. Nursing borrows and uses theories from other disciplines. An example of a non-nursing theory is Maslow's Hierarchy of Basic Human Needs.

    ❑ True

    ❑ False

14. In a conversation with two nurse colleagues, you hear a discussion about the scope of practice of the various helping disciplines. When discussing the difference between medicine and nursing, Nurse A says medicine and nursing share the same metaparadigm, citing that nurses carry out doctors' orders. Nurse B states that the metaparadigm of nursing is broader than that of medicine. Which of these nurses represents the perspective aligned with current nursing theory and practice?

    a. Nurse A

    b. Nurse B

15. The concept of homeostasis becomes obsolete when considering the theory of which of the following theorists?

    a. Jean Watson

    b. Dorothea Orem

    c. Martha Rogers

    d. Sr. Callista Roy

16. Nursing theory development began with the writings of Florence Nightingale in 1859. Place the following nursing theories in sequence from earliest development to most recent.

    _____ Jean Watson: The Philosophy and Science of Caring

    _____ Martha Rogers: A Science of Unitary Man

    _____ Virginia Henderson: The Nature of Nursing

    _____ Dorothea Orem: Self-Care Deficit Theory of Nursing

    _____ Rosemarie Parse: Man-Living-Health: A Theory of Nursing

    _____ Myra Levine: The Four Conservation Principles

    _____ Patricia Benner: From Novice to Expert

    _____ Madeline Leininger: Culture Care Diversity and Universality

    _____ Faye Abdellah: 21 Nursing Problems

17. Existentialism influenced the work of this early nursing theorist who focused her work on the human-to-human relationship and the meaning in experiences such as illness. Who was this theorist?

    a. Joyce Travelbee

    b. Faye Abdellah

    c. Myra Levine

    d. Patricia Benner

18. Which of the following nursing theories is consistent with the Simultaneity Paradigm?

    a. Martha Rogers

    b. Myra Levine

    c. Dorothea Orem

    d. Sr. Callista Roy

19. Mr. Hill, 38 years old, is a newly diagnosed diabetic. Since he is to be discharged tomorrow, you are reviewing aspects of his self-care regimen. You teach, reinforce, and ask for a demonstration of his ability to self-administer insulin injections. At the completion of the teaching session, he asks you to return later to review how to draw up insulin in a syringe. Which of the following theories would best describe the theoretical framework you will be operating through as you meet his self-care need?

    a. Orem's theory

    b. Watson's theory

    c. Levigne's theory

20. The discipline of nursing recommends that beginning practitioners learn one theory and apply it to all clinical situations.

    ❑ True

    ❑ False

Chapter 3 Nursing Education and Research

1. A factor believed to contribute to the decline in enrollments in all levels of nursing programs between 1995 and 1999 is

    a. a tightening of admission requirements within nursing programs.

    b. the increase in enrollments of second career individuals.

    c. the influence of managed care on the demand for nurses in the workforce.

    d. the proliferation of career opportunities for women.

2. The purpose of the State Board of Nursing in the process of the approval of schools of nursing is to

    a. set minimum practice criteria for nursing.

    b. ensure the safe practice of nursing by setting minimum educational requirements.

    c. accredit schools of nursing through a peer review process.

    d. ensure educational mobility for nurses who are prepared at the LPN or associate degree level for practice.

3. An LPN is prepared to provide care using basic skills in a variety of settings without RN supervision.

    ❑ True

    ❑ False

4. There is evidence that shows there is a relationship between health care quality and the educational level of the nursing staff within an agency.

    ❑ True

    ❑ False

5. Which of the following is considered the primary factor associated with the aging of the RN workforce?

    a. Nursing is a second career for many RNs.

    b. The numbers of nurses who leave nursing before midlife is on the increase.

    c. The number of younger people choosing nursing as a career is decreasing.

    d. None of the above.

6. Based on the Pew Health Professions Commission Report and *Nursing's Agenda for Health Care Reform*, graduates of nursing programs will

    a. have limited exposure to community-based health care experiences.

    b. be prepared within nursing practice environments where there is only access to nursing practice councils.

    c. have exposure to diverse client populations.

    d. have experiences with interdisciplinary practice.

7. It is estimated that the U.S. will have a shortage of nearly 114,000 full-time equivalent RNs by the year 2015.

    ❑ True

    ❑ False

8. Nurses will be increasingly employed by preferred-provider organizations in the future. A preferred-provider organization

    a. operates on a fee-for-service basis.

    b. always includes a primary provider who screens services.

    c. emphasizes the treatment of diseases vs. prevention of illness.

    d. is a type of managed care organization where members are limited to the providers in the organization.

9. The Pew Health Care Professionals' Competencies document emphasizes the need for health care professionals to continue to learn throughout their careers.

    ❑ True

    ❑ False

10. Half of the boards for nursing require continuing education units as a condition for relicensure. Does the evidence support the assertion that mandated continuing education guarantees continued competence?

    ❑ Yes

    ❑ No

11. Which of the following would likely lead to the implementation of evidence-based nursing practice?

    a. Efforts to change the behavior of the individual nurse

    b. The design of organizational systems that facilitate change

12. Which of the following type of research involves the systematic collection of numerical data, often under considerable control?

    a. Quantitative

    b. Qualitative

    c. Historical

13. Match the term in the left column with its definition from the right column.

    _____ hypothesis   a. Variation of a variable

    _____ independent variable   b. Statement of relationship between two variables

    _____ dependent variable   c. Abstraction inferred from situations or behaviors

    _____ construct   d. Outcome variable of interest

    _____ value   e. Controlled variable

14. When obtaining an informed consent from a client who is participating in a research study, the client is entitled to a full disclosure before signing a consent. This means that the client is informed about the nature of the study, the risks and benefits, as well as the right to refuse to participate.

    ❑ True

    ❑ False

15. Which of the following statements most accurately describes the role of the nurse without a graduate degree in the research process?

    a. Designs research projects

    b. Integrates research findings into care protocol changes

    c. Collects research data as part of a research team

    d. Acts as the principal investigator on a project

16. A research abstract is found at the beginning of a research article summarizing the purpose, methodology, findings, and conclusions of the study.

    ❑ True

    ❑ False

17. In which type of nursing program would a nurse practitioner student most likely be found?

    a. Associate Degree in Nursing

    b. Baccalaureate Degree in Nursing

    c. Diploma in Nursing

    d. Master's Degree in Nursing

18. You are searching the Web for information on clinical practive guidelines that are designed to improve the quality of care on your unit as well as reduce the costs for that care. Which of the following Web sites would be most appropriate to consult?

    a. *www.jacho.org*

    b. *www.nlnac.org*

    c. *www.aacn.nche.edu*

    d. *www.ahrg.gov/clinic/epc*

19. The National Institute of Nursing Research has as its major goal to conduct nursing research.

    ❑ True

    ❑ False

20. An article written by a nurse researcher is considered a

    a. primary source.

    b. secondary source.

    c. tertiary source.

Chapter 4   The Health Care Delivery System

1. Mrs. Becker has been admitted to a rehabilitation facility subsequent to a hip fracture repair at a local hospital. She is there for ambulation retraining and direct care during her recuperation. Which of the following types of care is this considered?

   a. Primary

   b. Secondary

   c. Tertiary

2. A physician who is reimbursed directly by an insurance company for services provided is being reimbursed by which of the following methods?

   a. Capitation

   b. Fee-for-service

   c. Single-payer reimbursement

3. In a prepaid (managed care) system, the goal of a health care provider such as a hospital would be to provide fewer services in order to save money.

   ❑ True

   ❑ False

4. In a landmark study by Mundinger et al. (2000), primary care outcomes were studied in patients treated by nurse practitioners or physicians 6 months and 1 year following initial appointment. Findings from this study would support which of the following statements?

   a. There is a significant difference in the treatment outcomes of patients treated by nurse practitioners or physicians.

   b. There is no difference in the treatment outcomes of patients treated by nurse practitioners or physicians.

   c. Clients reported preferring nurse practitioners over physicians as a health care provider.

   d. Clients reported preferring physicians over nurse practitioners as a health care provider.

5. Match the managed care model in the left column with its appropriate characteristic from the right column.

_____ HMO (Health Maintenance Organization)

a. Care must be delivered by the plan in order for clients to receive reimbursement

_____ PPO (Preferred Provider Organization)

b. Focus on care is on cost-effective treatment measures with quality outcomes

_____ EPO (Exclusive Provider Organization)

c. Members are limited to providers within the system

6. An issue that influences the quality of nursing care as increased nursing tasks are assigned to unlicensed assistive personnel (UAP) is the

a. length of time UAPs are trained.

b. character of the person filling the UAP role.

c. educational level of the nurse responsible for the care of the patient.

d. quality of data the nurse uses in clinical decision making.

7. Consider the phrase "The greatest good for the most people." The citizens of which country would agree that this is a guiding philosophy underpinning the health care system of their country?

a. United States

b. Canada

8. Which of the following health services is the most money spent on in the U.S.?

a. Medications

b. Nursing home care

c. Hospital care

d. Physicians' services

9. Which of the following groups spurred the movement toward cost containment of health care?

a. Physicians

b. Insurance companies

c. The business sector

d. The American Association of Retired Persons (AARP)

10. An oversupply of specialized health care providers plays a role in the increased cost of health care.

    ❑ True

    ❑ False

11. Which of the following represents the portion of RNs employed by hospitals?

    a. 50%

    b. 67%

    c. 76%

    d. 87%

12. The restructuring of hospitals is the result of cost-cutting measures by insurance companies, who use fee-for-service reimbursement structures.

    ❑ True

    ❑ False

13. The medical model has limited the role of nurses in the health care system.

    ❑ True

    ❑ False

14. Which of the following factors places the quality of hospital care at risk when hospitals restructure?

    a. Replacing brand name medications with generic drugs

    b. Replacing RNs with UAP

    c. Shortening the length of stay (LOS) for certain medical diagnoses

    d. Blending the roles of hospital workers into a multiskilled worker

15. Do you agree with the following statement? One factor that contributes to the demand for an increased number of nurses is the growing number of elderly people in the population.

    ❑ Yes

    ❑ No

16. What is the percentage of preschool children in this country who are not immunized?

    a. 15%

    b. 25%

    c. 35%

    d. 40%

17. In 1991 the nursing community put forth *Nursing's Agenda for Health Care Reform*. A cornerstone of this proposal is that

    a. all citizens must have access to health care services.

    b. health care services should be paid for by a single payer from public funds.

    c. health care must emphasize illness cure.

    d. integrated health systems must improve the continuity of care.

18. Which of the following statements would be accurate about nurse practitioner versus physician care?

    a. nurse practitioners charge more for service.

    b. nurse practitioners spend more time with their clients.

    c. nurse practitioners can independently diagnose and resolve 80% of primary health problems.

    d. nurse practitioners have prescriptive privileges in all states.

19. The Health Care Financing Administration (HCFA) funded CNOs to care for the indigent in the community.

    ❑ True

    ❑ False

20. Subacute care emphasizes

    a. high acuity care.

    b. home care.

    c. curative interventions.

    d. restorative interventions.

Chapter 5 Critical Thinking and the Nursing Process

1. Match the component of critical thinking on the left with its definition on the right.

    _____ mental operations

    a. The component of critical thinking that allows a person to question assumptions

    _____ knowledge

    b. The component of critical thinking that includes decision making

    _____ attitudes

    c. The component of critical thinking that requires facts or information

2. Indicate whether you agree or disagree with the following statement: Not all aspects of professional nursing practice involve critical thinking.

    ❑ Agree

    ❑ Disagree

3. Critical thinking in nursing practice requires a nurse to draw from a broad knowledge base in order to make sound clinical decisions. Which type of knowledge is used when a nurse recalls the facts of anatomy and physiology to solve a patient's clinical problem?

    a. Declarative

    b. Operative

4. Critical thinking plays a role in adaptation of the practicing nurse to the rapid pace of change occurring within the health care system.

    ❑ True

    ❑ False

5. Novice nurses develop clinical judgment as the length of time in nursing practice increases. Based on your understanding of critical thinking, which of the following statements is true about the development of clinical judgment?

    a. Clinical judgment develops at the same pace for every new nurse.

    b. New knowledge is unnecessary for clinical judgment to evolve.

    c. Exploration of alternative solutions to patient problems is not expected.

    d. An attitude of intellectual humility is the basis for questioning assumptions.

6. Several barriers to creative thinking have been identified in the literature. These include blocks such as comfort with the status quo, following tradition, operating with a rigid mindset, and going along with the majority opinion (groupthink). List two additional blocks that can interfere with creative thinking.

    1. _____

    2. _____

7. The *Standards for Nursing Practice*, first published in 1973, included the steps of the nursing process.

    ❑ True

    ❑ False

8. Match the type of nursing diagnosis from the left column with its definition from the right column.

    _____ actual diagnosis   a. A potential client problem

    _____ risk diagnosis   b. A situation where a problem could exist if no action is taken

    _____ possible diagnosis   c. An existing client problem

    _____ wellness diagnosis   d. Reflects a situation in which a nurse manages the client's health status with a physician

    _____ collaborative diagnosis   e. Reflects a desire of the client to improve health

9. Write in the type of assessment data, either Subjective data or Objective data, on the lines provided.

    _____ "My head hurts"

    _____ Wound circular, 1½ inches in diameter, redness around edges, no drainage present

    _____ "I hear voices telling me to hurt myself"

    _____ Unsteady gait, walked from bed to doorway of room

    _____ "I am feeling upset now, I can't concentrate"

    _____ Oxygen saturation 93% on room air

10. The nursing diagnosis, "Alteration in skin integrity related to immobility as manifested by stage 1 pressure ulcer on coccyx," is an example of which of the following nursing diagnoses?

    a. Risk diagnosis

    b. Possible diagnosis

    c. Wellness diagnosis

    d. Actual diagnosis

11. As nurse Kelley reviews the patient record for her assigned patient, she reads the physician's orders for a patient admitted to her unit with a diagnosis of pneumonia. Following this entry she reads down the list of treatments the physician has ordered. After she has assessed her patient, she begins to write the nursing care plan for this patient. She writes, "Ineffective airway clearance related to fatigue and weakness as manifested by inability to effectively cough and mobilize secretions." Reflect on the differences between the medical diagnosis and the nursing diagnosis. Which of the following statements is an accurate summary of the difference between a medical and a nursing diagnosis?

    a. The nursing diagnosis is determined by the medical diagnosis.

    b. The medical diagnosis is treated by the nurse.

    c. The nursing diagnosis reflects a human response to an actual problem.

    d. Only physicians can treat a pathophysiology.

12. Gordon's Functional Health Patterns is an example of a framework for organizing the collection of client data.

    ❏ True

    ❏ False

13. The nurse asks the question, "Are there any risk factors here that could affect the health of my client?" Which phase of the nursing process is the nurse using?

    a. Assessment

    b. Diagnosis

    c. Implementation

    d. Evaluation

14. An example of a priority nursing diagnosis is

    a. ineffective individual coping.

    b. risk for injury.

    c. risk for impaired skin integrity.

    d. sleep pattern disturbance.

15. Expected outcome statements must be realistic, have a time limit, and be

    a. clear.

    b. broad.

    c. measurable.

16. The implementation phase of the nursing process includes writing the nursing interventions for each nursing diagnosis on the care plan.

    ❑ True

    ❑ False

17. Which of the following activities does the implementation phase of the nursing process include?

    a. Giving care

    b. Recording patient responses

    c. Reporting significant changes

    d. All three answers

18. The major focus for the nurse in the evaluation phase of the nursing process is to determine if the goals established for the client have been met.

    ❑ True

    ❑ False

19. In which of the following aspects of the nursing process would a nurse use the critical thinking skill of differentiating between essential and trivial data to come to a thoughtful conclusion about a set of patient signs and symptoms?

    a. Assessment

    b. Diagnosis

    c. Outcome identification

    d. Implementation

20. The nursing process is a problem-solving process that uses the scientific method to identify problems and make decisions about client needs.

    ❑ True

    ❑ False

Chapter 6 Assessment

1. Your patient arrives in the emergency room with a chief complaint of substernal chest pain. Which type of assessment is most appropriate when greeting the patient?

    a. General

    b. Comprehensive

    c. Focal

    d. Ongoing

2. Which of the following aspects of a health history would a client most likely be reluctant to share with a nurse?

    a. Allergies

    b. Use of herbal preparations

    c. Previous hospitalizations

    d. Prescription medications

3. During the interview your patient states, "My right ear hurts off and on. Sometimes the pain is real sharp and I have to stop and wait for it to die down." Which of the following assessment techniques would you use to gather objective data?

    a. Palpation

    b. Inspection

    c. Percussion

    d. Auscultation

4. The nurse's aide comes to you and states Mrs. Phillips says she has chest pain. Mrs. Phillips was admitted today with severe coronary artery disease and has a standard Heparin infusing at 860 units per hour. Her lab CPK results show no elevations and her EKG results show no new changes. What will be your first action when you see Mrs. Phillips?

    a. Ask her to describe the location, duration, and character of the pain.

    b. Administer the sublingual nitroglycerin ordered by the physician.

    c. Tell her that the pain is the result of the cardiac catheterization she experienced two days ago.

    d. Ask her to describe, in detail, her cardiac history.

5. Match the best assessment technique from the right column for determining the assessment finding in the left column.

_____ abdominal distention	a. Auscultation
_____ adventitious breath sounds	b. Palpation
_____ circumoral pallor	c. Percussion
_____ lung tissue consolidation	d. Observation

6. A taxonomy of nursing diagnoses developed by the North American Nursing Diagnosis Association (NANDA) organizes client health care data into functional health patterns.

   ❑ True

   ❑ False

7. The telemetry technician states Mr. Slayer's heart rhythm and rate has just changed from normal sinus rhythm with a heart rate of 78 to atrial fibrillation with a heart rate of 124. On your way to assess Mr. Slayer's vital signs you obtain a sphygmomanometer. What important information will you need prior to performing this assessment?

   a. The most recent EKG results

   b. The most recent CPK results

   c. A review of his past physical illnesses

   d. The baseline vital signs

8. The type of assessment format used by a nurse has no impact on the nursing diagnosis statements generated from an assessment.

   ❑ True

   ❑ False

9. The best source of data about the client is the

   a. family.

   b. client's records.

   c. physician.

   d. client.

10. Mrs. Jones presents with an oral temperature of 100 degrees F. Her chief complaint is frequency and burning upon urination. You suspect that Mrs. Jones has a urinary tract infection. Which of the following assessments would validate your conclusion?

   a. Elevated WBC.

   b. Mrs. Jones is drinking large volumes of fluid.

   c. Elevated bacterial cell count of the urine.

   d. Mrs. Jones states, "When I have to go, I can't wait."

11. In what sequence would you expect to gather information about your hospitalized patients when you first begin your work shift?

_____ The medical record, the most recent lab work results

_____ The patient

_____ The care Kardex, care plan, assessment flow sheets

_____ The nurses' shift report about the patient

_____ The patient's family

_____ Health care personnel

12. During a physical examination the nurse encounters a symptom. The relevant data needed about a symptom would include location, character, intensity, timing, and the aggravating or alleviating factors.

❑ True

❑ False

13. Mr. Kamal is due to be discharged within four days. He will need assistance with activities of daily living and will need to have a prothrombin time drawn twice a week. Which of the following questions would best elicit information needed to plan for his discharge needs?

a. What kind of assistance will you need in order to go to the laboratory to have your blood tests done?

b. Will you need help at home?

c. Will a family member help you at home?

d. Do you have any assistive devices at home that will be of help to you?

14. You have just heard a report on your patient, Mrs. Smith, who has just returned from the OR after a cholescystectomy. She has an IV of D5 in 1/2 NS infusing at 100cc's per hour, O_2 at 4L per nasal cannula, an NG tube attached to continuous low wall suction, and a Foley catheter. She has been medicated for incisional discomfort with 10mg of Morphine Sulphate sc one hour ago. The report revealed that Mrs. Smith is slightly nauseated. Her husband is in the room with her. Which of the following assessments is priority upon entering the room?

a. The position of the siderails

b. Assessment of the wound for drainage

c. Check to see if the oxygen is set at the proper flow rate

d. The temperature of the room

15. The purpose of the physical examination is to verify and expand upon data obtained through the interview.

    ❑ True

    ❑ False

16. When interviewing the client, nurses must always elicit information about allergies.

    ❑ True

    ❑ False

17. Mr. Hays will be discharged on Digoxin 0.25mg PO q am. You are planning to discuss this medication with him. After reviewing nursing considerations for this medication, select the interview question that would be most helpful in planning for his needs.

    a. If your pulse is less than 50 beats per minute, what will you do?

    b. Where does this drug act on the body?

    c. Do you know what the side effects of Digoxin are?

18. Mr. Daniels has just arrived on your unit to undergo surgery the next morning. You need to interview him in order to complete your nursing assessment. His roommate has several noisy visitors and the TV is on. Which of the following actions could you take in order to accomplish the interview?

    a. Close the curtain to provide privacy.

    b. Ask his roommate to turn down the volume of the TV.

    c. Escort Mr. Daniels to a private, quiet space if a suitable room is available.

    d. All of the listed actions.

    e. None of the listed actions.

19. Within the introduction phase of the interview, the nurse and the client establish the goal(s) for the interaction.

    ❑ True

    ❑ False

20. Which of the following assessment formats is designed to document assessment data obtained from residents of a long-term care facility?

    a. The Sickness Impact Profile

    b. The Body Systems Model

    c. The Minimum Data Set

    d. Maslow's Hierarchy of Needs

Chapter 7   Nursing Diagnosis

1. There are similarities and differences between medical and nursing diagnoses. Which of the following is unique to the process of establishing a nursing diagnosis?

   a. The focus is on human responses to health problems.

   b. The diagnostic process is creative and organized.

   c. Assessment data is only collected and analyzed prior to the establishment of the diagnosis.

   d. It is legally sanctioned for the profession.

2. Nursing diagnosis is the third step in the nursing process.

   ❏ True

   ❏ False

3. Which of the following is best defined by the statement, "a clinical judgment about an individual, family, or community response to actual and potential health problems/life processes?"

   a. Nursing diagnosis

   b. Medical diagnosis

   c. Collaborative problem

   d. Independent problem

4. Nursing diagnosis *originally* appeared in nursing literature after the first National Conference for the Classification of Nursing Diagnoses convened in 1973.

   ❏ True

   ❏ False

5. The first nursing diagnosis conference in 1973 began to identify, develop, and place nursing diagnoses in a taxonomy. Which of the following statements is correct about the nursing diagnosis taxonomy?

   a. It is a list of nursing diagnoses.

   b. It is a classification of human responses.

   c. It is a complete list of all possible diagnoses.

   d. Each nursing diagnosis has been validated using medical diagnoses as a standard.

6. Consider the following nursing diagnosis: *Ineffective Airway Clearance R/T fatigue as evidenced by dyspnea at rest*. Which portion represents the etiology for this diagnosis?

   a. Ineffective airway clearance

   b. Fatigue

   c. Dyspnea at rest

7. List one of the two syndrome diagnoses accepted by NANDA.

   _____

8. A "risk" diagnosis contains three parts in the diagnostic statement.
   ❑ True
   ❑ False

9. Which of the following type of nursing diagnosis identifies the individual or aggregate condition or state that may be enhanced by health-promoting activities?

   a. Actual

   b. Risk

   c. Wellness

   d. Syndrome

10. List in sequence the steps in developing a nursing diagnosis.

_____ Data is clustered.

_____ The first part of the diagnosis is written (diagnostic label).

_____ Data cues are interpreted and assigned meaning.

_____ Related to (R/T) factors are identified and attached to the diagnosis.

_____ Data cues are identified from client data.

_____ Data cues are validated.

_____ A list of nursing diagnoses is consulted.

11. Consider the nursing diagnosis *Acute Pain R/T pain from incision*. Which of the following statements identifies the error in this nursing diagnosis?

   a. It is saying the same thing twice.

   b. It is using a medical diagnosis in the nursing diagnosis.

   c. It is a judgmental statement.

   d. It should have been written as a one-part nursing diagnosis.

12. Which of the following would be an appropriate nursing diagnosis for an adult who is dyspneic upon exertion, has an O_2 saturation of 88%, and has crackles in both lung bases? Vital signs are as follows: BP 106/70, P 98, R 32 (at rest), T 101.2°F.

   a. Risk for Respiratory Dysfunction

   b. Risk for Ineffective Airway Clearance

   c. Impaired Gas Exchange

   d. Impaired Airway Clearance

13. Which of the following wellness nursing diagnoses is written correctly?

   a. Readiness for Enhanced Spiritual Well-being

   b. Enhanced Spiritual Well-being

   c. Readiness for Spiritual Well-being

   d. Readiness for Enhanced Spiritual Well-being R/T religion seeking behavior

14. Consider the following assessment data. Mrs. Cho is 68 years old, with a medical diagnosis of arthritis and congestive heart failure (CHF). She states she eats very little and tries to adhere to her fluid restriction. She has not had a BM in two days. She becomes short of breath when she climbs the stairs at home. Her vital signs are as follows: BP 136/80, P 102, R 20, T 99.2°F. Which of the following is an accurate nursing diagnosis?

    a. Deficient Fluid Volume R/T fluid restriction

    b. Constipation R/T poor nutritional state

    c. Ineffective Breathing Pattern R/T congestive heart failure

    d. None of the above

15. Would you agree that the following nursing diagnosis is correctly written? *Noncompliance with treatment regimen: client depressed R/T recent death of wife.*

    ❑ Yes

    ❑ No

16. Many hospitals are using interdisciplinary care plans to monitor patient outcomes. Which of the following rationale best explains the reason for novice nurses to know nursing diagnosis and nursing process?

    a. Nursing care plans assist beginning nursing practitioners in determining the best possible nursing actions and desired patient outcomes for individualized patient care.

    b. Knowledge of the nursing process, nursing diagnosis, and care planning assists the beginning nursing practitioner in understanding the discipline of nursing and how it relates to the care focus of other health care disciplines.

Chapter 8   Outcome Identification and Planning

1. Planning is the third step of the nursing process.
   - ❑ True
   - ❑ False

2. According to the ANA Standards, which of the following is a criterion for the development of client expected outcomes?

   a. The outcome must be documented in measurable terms.

   b. The outcome must be comprehensive.

   c. The outcome must be setting specific.

   d. The outcome must be approved by an outside reviewer.

3. Match the term in the left column with its definition from the right column.

   _____ initial planning   a. An expectation to be achieved in a few days or hours

   _____ ongoing planning   b. The plan developed for the client's care upon leaving the facility

   _____ discharge planning   c. The continuous updating of the client's plan of care

   _____ short-term goal   d. The plan developed as a result of the admission assessment

   _____ long-term goal   e. An expectation to be achieved in weeks or months

4. Prioritize the following nursing diagnoses from *high* to *low* priority.

   _____ Hyperthermia

   _____ Risk for impaired skin integrity

   _____ Spiritual distress

5. Mr. Butterworth has been hospitalized for three days. When you enter his room to do the daily assessment, he asks you if he could be shaved today, citing that he has been unshaven since his admission. Which of the following is the best response?

    a. "I'm sorry, I do not have time today to shave you."

    b. "I will see if I can fit this into your plan of care for today. Let me get back to you."

    c. "I understand your need to be shaved; it will make you feel better. I will see to it that you get a shave."

    d. "Is your wife coming in today? Possibly she can shave you."

6. Which of the following type of goal concentrates on the client's return to maximal functioning?

    a. Short-term goal

    b. Long-term goal

7. All goal statements must have written conditions under which the client should perform the task or skill.

    ❑ True

    ❑ False

8. Which of the following terms does *not* describe a goal statement?

    a. It is measurable.

    b. It is written in current or past tense.

    c. It specifies a time frame for the task accomplishment.

    d. It is realistic for the client.

9. Which of the following type of nursing order is "Teach the client the importance of adherence to a low-fat diet"?

    a. Health promotion

    b. Prevention

    c. Observation

    d. Treatment

10. Which of the following would be an example of a client need where the nurse would call a consultation?

    a. The client is immobile and at risk for a break in skin integrity.

    b. The client has a knowledge deficit regarding ambulation with crutches on a flat surface as well as climbing stairs.

    c. The client has a Foley catheter and a primary IV infusing and is at risk for infection.

    d. The client is confused and frail with a history of falls and is at risk for injury.

11. In the following goal statement, which portion is the *task statement?* "The client will ambulate the entire length of the hallway three times by Friday."

    a. The client

    b. Will ambulate

    c. The entire length of the hallway

    d. By Friday

12. Consider the following client goal statement written for a client experiencing a knowledge deficit: "The client will know the reason for taking his medication before discharge." Is this goal acceptable?

    ❑ Yes

    ❑ No

13. Consider the goal statement, "The client will ambulate the entire length of the hallway three times a day with the use of a walker." Does this goal statement include a set of conditions by which the client will accomplish the goal?

    ❑ Yes

    ❑ No

14. The nursing profession can demonstrate a simple and straightforward way to link nursing interventions and client outcomes.

    ❑ True

    ❑ False

15. Consider the following nursing order: "10/21/00 At first sign of chest pain, instruct client to relax and discontinue activity. Mary Smith R.N." Is this acceptable as a nursing order?

    ❑ Yes

    ❑ No

16. Mrs. Langly is a 45-year-old client who has a history of diabetes, end-stage renal disease, and peripheral vascular disease. She was admitted to your unit for unstable blood levels of BUN, creatinine, and glucose. Which of the following goals would be appropriate for Mrs. Langly?

    a. The patient will plan a low-protein, 1800 calorie diabetic diet for 48 hours by Friday.

    b. The patient will demonstrate effective coping by discharge.

    c. The patient will be able to plan for an appropriate diet by Thursday.

    d. The patient will know why it is important to follow a diet by discharge.

17. When standardized nursing care plans are used in health care institutions, it is expected that the care plan will be individualized to meet client needs.

    ❑ True

    ❑ False

18. Consider the following nursing diagnosis for a one-day post-op client: *Risk for Infection R/T surgical incision*. Which of the following interventions would be appropriate for this nursing diagnosis?

    a. Assess wound for signs of redness or drainage q shift.

    b. Assess IV site for inflammation or infiltration.

    c. Change steri strips q shift, assess wound.

    d. Monitor pulse rate q 4h.

19. Consider the following nursing diagnosis for a patient who is on bedrest: *Risk for Altered Respiratory Function R/T stasis of secretions secondary to immobility*. Which of the following nursing interventions on the care plan was derived from the etiological portion of the nursing diagnostic statement?

    a. Offer the patient a back rub q shift.

    b. Encourage patient to do leg exercises q 2h.

    c. Assist patient to turn, deep breathe, and cough q 2h.

    d. Suction oral secretions PRN.

20. Which of the following system of standardized nursing language provides a basis to measure the effects of nursing practice on client outcomes?

    a. NIC

    b. NOC

    c. NANDA

Chapter 9 Implementation

1. At the beginning of a work shift a nurse establishes a shift worksheet considering patient care priorities. Which of the following would be placed on the shift worksheet first?

   a. Medication administration

   b. Patient assessments

   c. Care plan reviews

   d. Vital sign measurements

2. The transfer of tasks to an individual who is competent in performing these tasks is called

   a. delegation.

   b. management.

   c. validation.

   d. task segmentation.

3. Match the type of nursing management system in the left column with its definition in the right column.

   _____ functional nursing   a. The RN is the leader, LPNs care for acutely ill clients, nursing assistants serve trays and assist with ADLs

   _____ team nursing   b. RN assumes responsibility for client care and coordination of care regardless of the location of the client

   _____ primary nursing   c. Caregivers are assigned to a segment of the client care unit

   _____ modular nursing   d. Care is divided into tasks and each person assumes a task

   _____ case management   e. RN assumes responsibility for total client care

4. Which of the following care management systems is the most costly to maintain?

   a. Team nursing

   b. Modular care

   c. Case management

   d. Primary nursing

5. Which of the following statements is true about nursing interventions? They are

    a. actions that help clients achieve goals.

    b. written broadly, not specifically.

    c. exclusively dependent on physicians' orders.

    d. written as a goal statement.

6. Which of the following would *not* be a nursing intervention?

    a. Performing a thoracentesis

    b. Assisting with ADLs

    c. Discharge planning

    d. Drawing blood from a central line catheter

7. Which of the following is considered an example of a standing physician's order?

    a. A protocol for indwelling urinary catheter care

    b. Hemoglobin and hematocrit two days postpartum on all postpartum patients

    c. The procedure for the flush of peripherally inserted central line catheters

    d. A skin care protocol for a client who is immobile

8. Your instructor asks you for the rationale underlying the nursing intervention you have selected for a nursing diagnosis. Which of the following best describes a rationale?

    a. Theory

    b. Pathophysiological condition

    c. Fundamental principle

    d. Nursing measure

9. The standardized nursing language that offers the profession of nursing the potential for direct reimbursement of services is

    a. NIC.

    b. NOC.

    c. NANDA.

    d. ANA.

10. Clients have the right to refuse any intervention.

    ❏ True

    ❏ False

11. You are to administer an IV medication. Your patient has total parenteral nutrition (TPN), lipids, and a minibag of potassium (KC1) supplement infusing through separate IV lines. After preparing the IV medication you enter the patient's room and are unsure which IV line to use to administer the medication. What should you do?

    a. Call the pharmacy for help.

    b. Ask a fellow student nurse for an opinion.

    c. Seek the assistance of the staff nurse assigned to your patient.

    d. Use the IV line that is infusing the TPN.

12. The class of nursing interventions Electrolyte and Acid-Base Balance falls into which of the following domains of the Nursing Intervention Classification?

    a. Physiological: Basic

    b. Physiological: Complex

    c. Safety

    d. Health System

13. Discharge planning begins at the time of admission to a health care facility.

    ❑ True

    ❑ False

14. Which of the following nursing interventions is considered a skilled therapeutic intervention?

    a. Assisting a patient to ambulate with a walker

    b. Feeding a patient who has difficulty swallowing

    c. Bathing a patient who is confused

    d. Administering a medication to a patient who is hypertensive

15. It has been documented in the nursing literature that it is possible to reduce the occurrence of falls in the elderly through the use of nursing interventions.

    ❑ True

    ❑ False

16. Which of the following is expected of a nurse after carrying out a nursing intervention?

    a. Notifying the physician of completion of the intervention

    b. Explaining to the client the reason for the intervention

    c. Reassessing the client

17. Which of the following would create an opportunity for the nurse to teach a client?

    a. Medication administration

    b. Vital sign measurement

    c. Changing a wound dressing

    d. All of the above

18. When a task is delegated, the role of the nurse is to

    a. validate the skill level of the care provider.

    b. assume the task was completed as expected.

    c. allow the care provider independence during task completion.

19. During a shift report the nurse would state the assessment data and indicate any changes in the patient assessment from the previous shift.

    ❑ True

    ❑ False

20. Indicate whether you agree or disagree with the following statement: When documenting the results of a nursing intervention, it is desirable to include a description of the patient's response.

    ❑ Agree

    ❑ Disagree

Chapter 10 Evaluation

1. Check all of the following behaviors that apply to the evaluation of nursing care.

   ____a. Establishing the initial database for a client as a result of the admission assessment

   ____b. Juxtaposing the client's response against an expected outcome

   ____c. Inviting the parents of a pediatric client to discuss the progress of their child toward an expected outcome

   ____d. Interpreting a cardiac rhythm strip

   ____e. Determining whether an objective on the care plan was achieved by the client

   ____f. Asking the client what he or she would like to achieve as an outcome of treatment

2. Which of the following outcomes would you expect as a result of a nursing audit?

   a. Revision of the facility mission and philosophy statement

   b. Revision to the standards of care related to the prevention of falls

   c. Revision to the care plan of an individual client

   d. Revision of the job description of the unlicensed assistive personnel (UAP)

3. In which of the following phases of the nursing process is the evaluation process reflected?

   a. Assessment and Implementation

   b. Assessment and Diagnosis

   c. Outcome identification and Implementation

   d. Assessment, Diagnosis, Planning, and Implementation

4. You review the RN staff nurse job description at Mercy Hospital for accuracy, keeping in mind that the establishment of job descriptions is one mechanism the hospital uses to deliver quality outcomes. Which of the following describes the type of evaluation you are conducting?

   a. Structural

   b. Process

   c. Outcome

5. Which of the following evaluation methods reflects a process evaluation?

   a. The assistant manager asks you to review the patient records of the last 10 patients discharged for documentation of patient response to analgesics administered.

   b. The division director asks you to make rounds on all the patient care units to see if the nursing policies are easily accessible.

   c. The evening supervisor asks you to analyze the staffing patterns for evening shift to determine if staffing is adequate to meet the acuity needs of patients.

   d. The case manager for your patient asks you to determine if the patient's discharge goal related to knowledge deficit has been met.

6. Indicate whether you agree or disagree with the following statement: There are practice settings where nurses are not expected to evaluate client care.

   ❑ Agree

   ❑ Disagree

7. Which of the following would you monitor as an indicator of quality care?

   a. The level of your patients' functionality at the time of discharge

   b. The satisfaction of the physicians on your unit with the nursing care delivered at your facility

   c. The results of the client satisfaction survey that pertain to you unit

   d. The level of client comorbidity at the time of admission to your unit

8. During rounds, Mrs. Jones's physician asks you if Mrs. Jones has met the expected outcome of ambulating around the unit four times a day with minimal assistance. What primary data source would you consult before you answer the physician?

   a. The patient record

   b. The family

   c. The UAP

   d. The patient

9. You determine that your client has not met an expected outcome. What action do you take?

   a. Call a meeting of the interdisciplinary team.

   b. Ask the client why the goal was not accomplished.

   c. Call for a nursing consultation.

   d. Review and revise the care plan.

10. In the ANA Standard VI: Evaluation, the standard includes a statement that the client, significant others, and health care providers are involved in the evaluation process.

    ❑ True

    ❑ False

11. Evaluation is based primarily on

    a. information retrieval and documentation.

    b. observation and communication.

    c. effective use of the nursing process.

    d. delivery of nursing care and analysis of client goals.

12. The accountability of nurses for their practice plays a limited role in the quality of health care delivery.

    ❑ True

    ❑ False

13. An aspect of evaluation that provides a basis for autonomy and self-governance for nursing practice is

    a. the application of agency standards.

    b. the peer evaluation process.

    c. multidisciplinary collaboration.

    d. the application of union rules to nursing practice.

Chapter 11   Nursing, Healing, and Caring

1. Of the following behaviors, check which behaviors display a nurse caring for a client.

    ____a. Responding in a compassionate manner

    ____b. Anticipating a client need

    ____c. Responding to a client who is fearful

    ____d   Calling a client "hun" or "dearie"

    ____e. Providing preprocedural information

    ____f. Delay in answering a call light

    ____g. Focusing attention on the treatment, not on the client

2. Care that is humanistic, emphasizing the client's individuality, counteracts which of the following processes that could occur during hospitalization?

    a. Depersonalization

    b. Oppression

    c. Empowerment

    d. Adaptation

3. It is evident that very few caring behaviors cross cultures.

    ❏ True

    ❏ False

4. Write in the appropriate relationship type, Social or Therapeutic, on the lines provided.

    _____ is spontaneous

    _____ communication is planned

    _____ is based on mutual interests

    _____ each participant expects to be liked by the other

    _____ has clear boundaries

5. Would you agree or disagree with the following statement?: Problem solving is a major component of caring.

   ❑ Agree

   ❑ Disagree

6. In which of the following phases of the nurse–client relationship would the nurse expect the client to exhibit testing behaviors?

   a. Orientation

   b. Working

   c. Termination

7. A nurse answers the questions of a new mother regarding newborn care at home. In which of the following phases of the nurse–client relationship would this occur?

   a. Orientation

   b. Working

   c. Termination

8. It is the responsibility of the nurse to protect client confidentiality at all times.

   ❑ True

   ❑ False

9. Match the characteristic of therapeutic relationships in the left column with its definition from the right column.

   _____ catharsis   a. A connection between two people based on mutual trust

   _____ rapport   b. The process of "getting things off one's chest"

   _____ empathy   c. Acting on the behalf of the client

   _____ advocacy   d. The perception of the situation as the client perceives it

10. **Patient** (admitted for surgery): "I found out three days ago that I have this cancer in my breast and now the doctor says my breast has to be removed."

    Nurse: "That's too bad, I'm sorry this is happening to you."

    Of which of the following terms is this interaction an example?

    a. Empathy

    b. Sympathy

11. The therapeutic tool of the nurse where the nurse remains physically with the patient is referred to as _____.

12. Which of the following behaviors by a nurse would foster trust?

    a. Hurriedly checking an IV site and administering the IV medication

    b. Sitting down and making frequent eye contact during a client interview

    c. Changing a client's dressing while talking to a coworker

    d. Not divulging the client's blood pressure when the client asks for this information

13. The use of humor is appropriate in all nurse–client relationships.

    ❑ True

    ❑ False

14. Match the essential behavior of trust in the left column with an example of it from the right column.

    _____ honesty   a. Providing privacy

    _____ consistency   b. Following through on a promise

    _____ respect   c. Maintaining confidentiality

15. Nurses view relieving a patient's pain and anxiety as a major aspect of their caring role.

    ❑ True

    ❑ False

16. In which of the following roles is a nurse functioning when a client is helped to increase coping skills?

    a. Caregiver

    b. Teacher

    c. Resource person

    d. Counselor

Chapter 12 Therapeutic Communication

1. The purpose of communication is to

   a. convey information to others.

   b. establish and maintain meaningful relationships.

   c. assess clients.

   d. provide feedback to the sender of a message.

2. Match the component of the communication process in the left column with the definition of the term in the right column.

   _____ sender   a. Can be verbal or nonverbal

   _____ message   b. Generates messages

   _____ channel   c. Received as a reaction to a message

   _____ receiver   d. Intercepts messages

   _____ feedback   e. Can be auditory, visual, or kinesthetic

3. Match the type of personal space in the left column with a therapeutic example from the right column.

   _____ intimate distance   a. Teaching a diabetic education class

   _____ personal distance   b. Giving an injection

   _____ social distance   c. Client demonstration of tube feeding

4. Which of the following best explains the importance of validating communication?

   a. Many clients with whom a nurse interacts are cognitively impaired.

   b. It assists a client with clarifying thoughts.

   c. Eye contact does not send the same message from culture to culture.

   d. Perceptions influence the interpretation of a message.

5. Self-talk can interfere with communicating with others.

   ❏ True

   ❏ False

6. Which of the following is a characteristic of effective feedback? It is

   a. general vs. specific.

   b. independent of time.

   c. best delivered in a small-group setting.

   d. clear and unambiguous.

7. When assessing a client's communication, the nurse assesses for congruence between the verbal and nonverbal messages the patient conveys. What does congruence mean?

   a. The verbal and nonverbal messages match.

   b. The verbal and nonverbal messages do not match.

   c. The client is predominantly communicating using nonverbal cues.

   d. The client is predominantly using words to communicate.

8. You walk into Ms. Grady's room and observe that her posture is slumped and she looks disheveled. Would you agree that this nonverbal behavior means that she is depressed?

   ❑ Yes

   ❑ No

9. Match the type of group in the left column with the example from the right column.

   _____ self-help group   a. Committee to study needlestick injuries

   _____ therapeutic group   b. Alcoholics Anonymous

   _____ therapy group   c. Eating disorders group

   _____ task group   d. Lifestyle change group (to reverse coronary artery disease)

10. The physical appearance of a nurse is not important to the nurse–client communication.

   ❑ True

   ❑ False

11. Match the principle of therapeutic interactions in the left column with its rationale in the right column.

_____ timeliness

_____ privacy

_____ comfort

_____ client focus

_____ focus on client feelings

_____ awareness of nurse's anxiety

a. Anxiety influences interaction

b. Allows the client to discuss problems and needs

c. Provides for confidentiality

d. Allows for discussion about troublesome events or situations

e. Ensures the client's attention during the interview

f. Eliminates distractions

12. Which of the following behaviors of a nurse indicates to a client that the nurse is actively listening?

a. The nurse's lips are pursed.

b. The nurse is shifting around in the chair.

c. The nurse makes eye contact.

d. The nurse changes the subject frequently.

13. Would you agree that when conveying an empathetic response to a client, the emotional distance is decreased between the client and the nurse?

❑ Yes

❑ No

14. A nurse says, "Tell me about what concerns you most today." This request is an example of which of the following communication techniques?

a. Broad opening statement

b. Reflection

c. Focusing

d. Restating

15. **Patient:** "I feel so angry when my husband refuses to come to the hospital and stay with me."

Nurse: "Why do you feel this way?"

Is this a therapeutic response?

❑ Yes

❑ No

16. **Client**: "My son has had this rash for nine months. The doctor gave me this anti-itch cream; it helps, but look, the rash is spreading. I don't know what to do anymore."

    Nurse: "You sound frustrated with this situation."

    The nurse's response is an example of which of the following communication techniques?

    a. Focusing

    b. Exploring

    c. Restating

    d. Reflection

17. **Patient**: "My surgery was five days ago. I notice that the other patients who have had the same kind of surgery aren't having the breathing problems that I am having. Should I worry about this?"

    Which of the following responses would be most therapeutic?

    a. "I'm sure everything will work out. Not everyone recovers at the same rate."

    b. "No, I don't think so."

    c. "Let me look at your chart. I'll be right back. Maybe the physician has written something in the chart that will be of help."

    d. "Can you tell me more about your breathing problems? Describe them for me."

18. A nurse assists a client with ambulation by holding onto the client. This action communicates caring through the kinesthetic communication channel.

    ❏ True

    ❏ False

19. You observe your patient, an insulin-dependent diabetic, eat several chocolates from a box of candy a guest has left at the bedside. The patient notices you, looks embarrassed, and states, "It's been a long time since I've had any candy. My, they tasted good." Which of the following responses by the nurse is most helpful?

    a. "You know you shouldn't be eating those. They are not good for you."

    b. "You did the right thing by stopping. Candy is bad for you."

    c. "I noticed you seemed embarrassed when you saw me. Would you like to talk about how you are feeling?"

    d. "Would you like to review what foods are part of your diabetic diet?"

20. Men are better decoders of nonverbal cues than women.

    ❏ True

    ❏ False

21. You observe a fellow student communicate with his patient, who does not speak English. The patient relies on her daughter to translate. The student nurse directs his communication to the patient's daughter. Would you agree that this student's behavior is appropriate?

    ❑ Yes

    ❑ No

22. Mrs. Alfonse, 80 years old, was admitted to your long-term care facility two days ago from the local hospital status post left-sided CVA. She cannot ambulate and has to be lifted to a chair. She has a pressure ulcer on her sacrum. As you re-dress it she states, "I can't believe I'm in a nursing home. What's going to become of me? I can't walk, I can barely feed myself, and I already have a sore on my bottom." Which of the following statements reflects a therapeutic response?

    a. "I'll leave a message for your doctor, so when she comes in she can talk about your progress."

    b. "That sounds like you are depressed. We can talk about it later."

    c. "You sound afraid for the future. If you want to talk about it, I would like to hear about it."

    d. "Let me finish with this dressing and I'll get you fixed up and you will feel better."

23. Mr. Bogardus is scheduled for surgery tomorrow to have a heart valve replaced. He asks, "How do people do after this kind of surgery?" The nurse replies, "Most people do well. We have a very low rate of complication after heart valve surgery at this hospital." Is the reply therapeutic?

    ❑ Yes

    ❑ No

24. Which of the following skills is the foundation of therapeutic communication?

    a. Active listening

    b. Validation

    c. Interviewing

    d. Restating

25. Should you assume an unconscious client can hear you?

    ❑ Yes

    ❑ No

Chapter 13   Client Education

1. Which of the following statements indicates that a client is ready to learn about diabetes? The client states:

    a. "I will go to the diabetes class tomorrow."

    b. "Tell my wife about my diabetes. She is better at remembering that sort of stuff."

    c. "My doctor tells me I should learn more about the foods I should or should not eat."

    d. "Show me how to inject myself with insulin."

2. Mr. Graves has received his learning materials about caring for himself at home after his surgery. Which of the following methods would best determine that he understands how to care for his incision?

    a. You ask him if he has read the booklet.

    b. You ask him to explain how to care for his incision.

    c. You show him how to cleanse the incision and apply a dressing.

    d. You ask his wife if Mr. Graves understands how to care for his incision.

3. The principles of learning theory say that feedback is most effective when it is

    a. positive and immediate.

    b. negative and immediate.

    c. positive and delayed.

    d. negative and delayed.

4. A client learns how to self-catheterize. Which of the following domains of learning does this represent?

    a. Cognitive

    b. Affective

    c. Psychomotor

5. Organizing content from the simple to the complex makes the learning process proceed in a user-friendly direction. Which of the following learning theorists would subscribe to this principle?

    a. Ivan Pavlov

    b. John Dewey

    c. Jerome Bruner

    d. Robert Gagne

6. Research demonstrates that there is a tight link between what clients determine as priority learning needs and what health care providers determine as learning needs.

    ❑ True

    ❑ False

7. Match the age group in the left column with the appropriate teaching strategy for that age group from the right column.

_____	children	a.	Play imitation
_____	adolescents	b.	Teach the client during the time of day in which the client is better able to concentrate
_____	middle-aged adults	c.	Identify and build on positive qualities
_____	older adults	d.	Prepare print-based material at an appropriate reading skill level

8. Ms. Norcross has been diagnosed with hypertension. During her office visit the physician refers her to you for diet and medication counseling. Which of the following phases of care does this activity reflect?

    a. Primary

    b. Secondary

    c. Tertiary

9. A nurse considers the who, what, when, and where of patient teaching in which of the following phases of the teaching-learning process?

    a. Assessment

    b. Identification of learning needs

    c. Planning

    d. Implementation

10. Mr. Canton is being discharged from the hospital in two days. He was admitted for a hypertensive crisis episode due to noncompliance with his prescribed medication regime. Which of the following assessments is a priority in order to determine his discharge planning needs?

    a. His ability to purchase his medications

    b. The cleanliness of his home

    c. The availability of someone to help with his care

    d. The availability of a hypertension education group in his immediate area

11. Ms. Chalahan was admitted this morning with a diagnosis of generalized anxiety disorder. Ms. Chalahan established the following discharge goal with her therapy team: "I will develop and use coping skills to manage my anxiety." Which of the following statements will determine that Ms. Chalahan has met her goal?

    a. "I can cope with my stressors."

    b. "My anxiety level is manageable at a level of 2 on a scale of 1–5."

    c. "I know what stress management techniques I need to learn in order to cope."

    d. "My nurse will tell me when I need to calm down."

12. Everyone who receives health care services has some need for learning.

    ❑ True

    ❑ False

13. Mr. Greyson, admitted for a bleeding ulcer, has a learning outcome on his patient teaching protocol that states, "Patient will verbalize signs and symptoms of GI bleeding and report to nurse or MD." After discussing the signs and symptoms of GI bleeding with Mr. Greyson, which of the following recordings reflect that the standard for documentation has been met for patient teaching?

    a. Mr. Greyson was taught the signs and symptoms of GI bleeding and seemed to understand the information.

    b. Mr. Greyson was read the materials that described the signs and symptoms of GI bleeding. He said he would take the information home with him.

    c. Mr. Greyson asked about the signs and symptoms of GI bleeding, questions were answered, and he seemed satisfied with the information.

    d. Mr. Greyson was given written information about the signs and symptoms of GI bleeding. It was reviewed with him. Correct responses were given to follow-up questions.

14. How would you determine the priority learning need(s) of your assigned client?

    a. Review the list of client learning outcomes.

    b. Conduct a comprehensive learning needs assessment.

    c. Identify the actual and potential learning needs and address the actual need first.

    d. Ask the client if there are any questions you can answer.

15. Joey, age 4, has fallen and cut his eyebrow. The physician in your clinic has just finished suturing the laceration. Joey continues to sob and his mother repeats, "It's my fault, if I had only watched him more closely this wouldn't have happened." Before Joey is discharged you must review the discharge instructions with his mother. Is this a good time to approach Joey's mother with the discharge instructions?

    ❏ Yes

    ❏ No

16. A client's concept of self-efficacy is linked to motivation to learn.

    ❏ True

    ❏ False

17. Which of the following learning goals is correctly stated?

    a. Mr. Jones will state the side effects of Digoxin.

    b. By his discharge date Mr. Saunders will be able to select from a list of foods those that contain Vitamin K and state which foods are to be avoided.

    c. At the time of admission for surgery, Ms. Barringer will have read her preoperative instructions.

    d. Within one week Mrs. Hanly will learn how to use her walker.

18. Does the Joint Commission for Accreditation of Healthcare Organizations mandate client teaching?

    ❏ Yes

    ❏ No

19. A peak in the effectiveness of teaching and depth of learning is called a _____.

20. It is important that nurses know the reading and comprehension abilities of their patients before using written materials in the education process. Which of the following ratios depicts the number of functionally illiterate Americans?

a. 1 in 3

b. 1 in 4

c. 1 in 5

d. 1 in 6

Chapter 14 Nursing and Complementary/Alternative Treatment Modalities

1. Ayurvedic medicine embraces the concept of *prana*. *Prana* is best thought of as a

    a. meditative practice.

    b. life force or energy.

    c. transport system for body energy.

2. The field of science that studies the relationship between the cognitive, affective, and physical aspects of humans is called

    a. neuroanatomy.

    b. psychoneuroimmunology.

    c. neurophysiology.

    d. psychobiology.

3. Which of the following groups of physiological responses reflects the benefits of meditation?

    a. Increased oxygen consumption, increased heart rate, and increased blood pressure

    b. Decreased oxygen consumption, decreased heart rate, and decreased blood pressure

    c. Alteration in immune system function, increased levels of lactic acid, and decreased blood pressure

    d. Alteration in immune system function, increased levels of lactic acid, and increased blood pressure

4. Which of the following perspectives on the practice of medicine would emphasize health maintenance and disease prevention through lifestyle choice?

    a. Alternative medicine

    b. Allopathic medicine

5. Which of the following statements best describes the goal of the nurse when the nurse serves as an instrument of healing? The goal is to

   a. provide therapeutic touch to clients when needed.

   b. dispense medicinal herbs useful for a wide variety of ailments.

   c. help the client draw upon inner resources for healing to occur.

   d. help the client access the life force energy in order to facilitate healing.

6. A 1998 survey found that 54% of U.S. adults used one or more complementary/alternative medicine (CAM) in the previous year. Based on the findings of this study, would you agree or disagree with the following statement? Over 50% of people who used CAM do not tell their primary care providers about the use of alternative health care approaches.

   ❑ Agree

   ❑ Disagree

7. Which of the following complementary/alternative interventions is considered a body-movement intervention?

   a. Tai chi

   b. Imagery

   c. Acupuncture

   d. Aromatherapy

8. Which of the following best describes the physiologic source of the relaxation response?

   a. Increased arousal of the sympathetic system

   b. Increased arousal of the parasympathetic system

   c. Suppression of the parasympathetic system

   d. Suppression of the sympathetic system

9. Sequence the following therapeutic touch (TT) phases in order from the beginning of an intervention to the end of an intervention.

   _____ Evaluation

   _____ Unruffling

   _____ Scanning

   _____ Centering

   _____ Balancing, rebalancing

10. In both therapeutic touch and healing touch, the practitioner uses centering before initiating treatment. Which of the following best describes the process of centering? Centering is

   a. a process of bringing body, mind, and emotions to a quiet, focused state of consciousness.

   b. a process of focusing attention on a client.

   c. a process whereby the emotional involvement between the practitioner and client is genuine and purposeful.

   d. a process whereby the practitioner directs energy toward the client.

11. The massage technique in which the whole hand is used to provide firm, gliding, even-pressured strokes is called

   a. effleurage.

   b. petrissage.

   c. tapotement.

   d. vibration.

12. Massage therapy is contraindicated for someone experiencing phlebitis.

   ❏ True

   ❏ False

13. Research has documented the effectiveness of therapeutic touch in the reduction of serum potassium in hyperkalemic states.

   ❏ True

   ❏ False

14. A client who chooses to follow a macrobiotic diet seeks foods containing macro-organic molecules.

   ❏ True

   ❏ False

15. Which of the following is a source of phytoestrogens?

   a. Green tea

   b. Tomatoes

   c. Onions

   d Soybeans

16. An unstable molecule that alters genetic codes and triggers the development of cancer cells is a(n)

    a. antioxidant.

    b. free radical.

    c. phytochemical.

    d. neuropeptide.

17. The herb Saint John's wort is believed to have medicinal value for the treatment of mild to moderate depression.

    ❏ True

    ❏ False

18. Which of the following herbal products, when combined with Coumadin, increases the risk of bleeding?

    a. Licorice root

    b. Danshen

    c. Belladonna

    d. Ginkgo biloba

19. It has been demonstrated that institutionalized clients exposed to pet therapy have improved socialization and mood and decreased blood pressure.

    ❏ True

    ❏ False

20. Yoga is an appropriate complementary therapy to use with preschoolers.

    ❏ True

    ❏ False

Chapter 15   Health, Holism, and the Individual

1. Match the term in the left column with its definition from the right column.

   _____ health

   a. A process through which a person seeks to maintain an equilibrium that promotes stability and comfort

   _____ illness

   b. The process by which a person adjusts to achieve homeostasis

   _____ wellness

   c. Functioning to one's maximum health potential

   _____ homeostasis

   d. Optimal level of functioning

   _____ adaptation

   e. Equilibrium among psychological, physiological, sociocultural, intellectual, and spiritual needs

   _____ high-level wellness

   f. Failure of adaptive responses that results in an impairment of functional abilities

2. You note that your client has unmet physiological and psychological needs. Which of the following unmet needs would be addressed as a priority?

   a. Physiological

   b. Psychological

3. Which of the following theoretical perspectives on health would a nurse be operating through when he or she assists a person with the use of health-promoting activities?

   a. Dunn

   b. Pender

   c. Bandura

   d. Rosenstock

4. List three nursing actions that can meet a patient's psychological need for security, a sense of belonging, and self-esteem.

   1. _____

   2. _____

   3. _____

5. Place the phases of the human sexual response in the proper sequence.

_____ Plateau

_____ Resolution

_____ Orgasm

_____ Excitement

6. Match the term in the left column with its definition from the right column.

_____ sexuality

a. The belief that one is psychologically of the sex opposite to his or her anatomic gender

_____ sex roles

b. The human characteristic that refers to all aspects of being male or female, including feelings, attitudes, beliefs, and behavior

_____ gender identity

c. Having an equal or almost equal preference for partners of either sex

_____ sexual orientation

d. How one views oneself as male or female in relationship to others

_____ heterosexuality

e. Culturally determined patterns of behavior associated with being male and female

_____ homosexuality

f. Sexual activity between two members of the same sex

_____ bisexuality

g. Sexual activity between a man and a woman

_____ transexuality

h. An individual's preference for expressing sexual feelings

7. A person with an *internal* locus of control feels like a victim.

❏ True

❏ False

8. Which of the following terms describes an individual's perception of his or her own ability to perform a certain task?

a. Empowerment

b. Self-efficacy

c. Self-concept

d. Self-esteem

9. Mrs. Evans recently learned that she has been diagnosed with lung cancer. She states, "Why me, why must it be me? I have taken such good care of myself. I don't know how I am going to cope with all of this. Nurse, what should I do?"

   Which of the following responses would best support Mrs. Evans's emotional and spiritual needs?

   a. "I will ask your physician to get a consult with the staff social worker."

   b. "Next time the hospital chaplain is here, I will ask him to stop by to see you."

   c. "Let me get your medications; you will feel better after you take them."

   d "Tell me more about your situation. I have a few minutes; I can stay and talk awhile."

10. Which of the following types of medications are associated with sexual dysfunction?

    a. Antihypertensives

    b. Antipyretics

    c. Antidiabetics

    d. Anticoagulants

11. Should *all* clients be assessed for sexual abuse?

    ❑ Yes

    ❑ No

12. An example of a health promotion activity is a client engaging in a cardiac rehabilitation program after suffering a myocardial infarction (heart attack).

    ❑ True

    ❑ False

13. Disease prevention occurs on a continuum. Which of the following is an example of *tertiary* prevention?

    a. A nurse conducts parenting classes at the local hospital.

    b. The local hospital offers blood pressure screening clinics once a month.

    c. A local health maintenance organization (HMO) offers stress management classes.

    d. A nurse works in a short-term rehabilitation facility assisting stroke patients to regain functional ability.

14. In order for a nurse to be an effective change agent when assisting clients to adopt a healthier lifestyle, which of the following would a nurse incorporate into the care plan?

    a. A standard, unmodified teaching plan for all clients

    b. The client's individual beliefs and motivations for change

    c. Regular appointments for a check-up

    d. Enroll the client in a wellness program

15. Which of the following is an example of an intervention that empowers the client?

    a. Linking a breastfeeding mother with La Leche League International

    b. Arranging for the spouse of a fully functioning client to manage and administer the client's medication in the home environment

    c. Feeding a client when the client is able to feed self

    d. Planning a bathing and grooming schedule for a functioning client

Chapter 16 Cultural Diversity

1. Match the term in the left column with its definition from the right column.

   _____ culture

   a. The dynamic and integrated structures of knowledge, beliefs, behaviors, ideas, values, habits, customs, languages, symbols, rituals, ceremonies, and practices unique to a particular group of people

   _____ ethnicity

   b. A group that constitutes less than the majority of the population

   _____ race

   c. A group of people who have experiences different from the larger culture or society that functionally unifies the group

   _____ stereotyping

   d. The group whose values prevail within a society

   _____ dominant culture

   e. A grouping of people based on biological similarities

   _____ minority group

   f. Labeling people based on cultural preconceptions

   _____ subculture

   g. A cultural group's perception of themselves

2. By the year 2050, less than 50% of the total U.S. population will be white.

   ❑ True

   ❑ False

3. There are six organizing factors nurses must consider when delivering culturally competent care: space, orientation to time, social organization, environmental control, biological variations, and _____.

4. Match the cultural group in the left column with the disorder most likely to affect the group from the right column.

   _____ African American

   a. Heart disease

   _____ Asian American

   b. Glaucoma

   _____ European American

   c. Lactose intolerance

   _____ Native American, Eskimo

   d. Sickle cell anemia

5. In which of the following cultural groups is eye contact considered a sign of disrespect?

   a. European American

   b. Native American

   c. Hispanic American

6. The *nuclear* family consists of the parents, children, and other relatives.

   ❏ True

   ❏ False

7. In which of the following cultures does the family assume greater importance than the individual?

   a. Gay

   b. Middle-class European American

   c. Hispanic

   d. Upper-class European American

8. According to the U.S. Department of Health and Human Services, a family of four with an annual income of $14,000 lives below the poverty line.

   ❏ True

   ❏ False

9. Which of the following best explains the purpose of the U.S. government WIC program?

   a. It provides destitute AIDS cases with supplemental income.

   b. It provides the homeless with shelter.

   c. It provides pregnant and breastfeeding mothers with supplemental food and other health services.

   d. It provides homeless children with food, shelter, and clothing.

10. Which of the following health problems would you expect to find among the homeless?

    a. Stroke

    b. Respiratory diseases

    c. Arthritis

    d. Keloid formation

11. Indicate whether you agree or disagree with the following statement: An increase in either income or education increases the likelihood of good health status across race and ethnic groups.

   ❑ Agree

   ❑ Disagree

12. Match the cultural group in the left column with its traditional healer from the right column.

   _____ African American   a. Herbalist

   _____ Asian American   b. Shaman

   _____ European American   c. Curandero

   _____ Hispanic American   d. "Community Mother"

   _____ Native American   e. Physician

13. In which of the following cultural groups would antihypertensives be administered in higher doses?

   a. African American

   b. Asian American

   c. Native American

   d. European American

14. Which of the following approaches is essential to the delivery of culturally sensitive care?

   a. Technical competence

   b. Detailed knowledge of the client's culture

   c. A nonjudgmental attitude

   d. Fluency in the client's native language

15. Fifty percent of the homeless people are on the streets because they have some form of mental illness or addiction.

   ❑ True

   ❑ False

Chapter *17* *The Life Cycle*

1. During each developmental stage of the life cycle, developmental tasks must be achieved. Which of the following phrases is the best example of the achievement of a developmental task?

   a. The normal physical development of a neonate from newborn to preschool age.

   b. An adolescent forms relationships with members of the opposite sex.

   c. A woman experiences breast tenderness and engorgement during the first trimester of pregnancy.

   d. An elderly man loses interest in sex due to decreased levels of testosterone in the blood.

2. Heredity, of all factors that influence growth and development, plays the most important role in determining a person's behavior.

   ❑ True

   ❑ False

3. Which of the following developed a theory of moral development based on studies of women?

   a. Gilligan

   b. Kohlberg

   c. Piaget

   d. Sullivan

4. Which of the following theorists postulated that an individual's unconscious processes are a motivator of behavior?

   a. Freud

   b. Piaget

   c. Kohlberg

   d. Gilligan

5. According to Erikson's stages of psychosocial development, which of the following stages of development would a person be in if the task to be achieved is to view one's life as meaningful and fulfilling?

    a. Identity vs. role diffusion

    b. Intimacy vs. isolation

    c. Generativity vs. stagnation

    d. Integrity vs. despair

6. Match Freud's psychosexual stage in the left column with its description from the right column.

    _____ oral

    _____ anal

    _____ phallic

    _____ latency

    _____ genital

    a. Emergence of sexual maturity, formation of relationships with potential sexual partners

    b. Management of anxiety by using mouth and tongue

    c. Quiet stage during which sexual energy is repressed and sexual development lies dormant

    d. Awareness of sex and genitalia

    e. Control of muscles, especially those controlling urination and defecation

7. If a fixation occurs during a stage of growth and development, a person progresses in a healthy manner through subsequent stages.

    ❑ True

    ❑ False

8. A major psychological task of neonates is to _____ with parents.

9. In which stage of Piaget's phases of cognitive development is the ability to see relationships and to do abstract thinking developed?

    a. Sensorimotor

    b. Preoperational

    c. Concrete operations

    d. Formal operations

10. At what age would you expect a child to form short simple sentences?

    a. 1 year

    b. 18 months

    c. 2 years

    d. 3 years

11. Place the following stages of faith, according to Fowler, in the proper sequence.

_____ Conjunctive faith

_____ Universalizing faith

_____ Intuitive-projective faith

_____ Mythical-literal faith

_____ Undifferentiated faith

_____ Individuative-reflective faith

_____ Synthetic-conventional faith

12. In which trimester of pregnancy is the fetus most susceptible to the effects of alcohol and other teratogenic substances?

   a. First

   b. Second

   c. Third

13. Breast milk and formula provide the same nutritional benefits for an infant.

   ❏ True

   ❏ False

14. Which of the following is the leading cause of death in young children?

   a. Suicide

   b. Respiratory disease

   c. Sports injuries

   d. Accidents

15. When teaching a preadolescent female about menstrual periods, which of the following statements would be accurate to relate?

   a. The average age of menarche is 10 years old.

   b. The menstrual cycle becomes regular after about 6–12 months.

   c. Approximately 40% of American females experience premenstrual syndrome.

   d. During the first few menstrual cycles, females do not ovulate.

16. In which of the following age groups are individuals at the highest risk for suicide?

    a. Preadolescent

    b. Adolescent

    c. Young adult

    d. Middle adult

17. George, a 16-year-old student, comes to the school nurse presenting with the following symptoms: urethitis, purulent discharge, urinary frequency, and inflammation of the epididymis. From which of the following STDs is George most likely suffering?

    a. Chlamydia

    b. Gonorrhea

    c. Genital warts

    d. Trichomoniasis

18. Which of the following would be appropriate to teach a middle-aged adult regarding physiological changes?

    a. Explain to men that enlargement of the prostate gland is common.

    b. Encourage a balance of exercise/activity and rest and sleep.

    c. Teach about fall precaution measures.

    d. Teach about the need for adequate calcium intake.

19. Which of the following would be the focus of a wellness program for middle-aged adults?

    a. Stress management

    b. Fall prevention

    c. Suicide prevention

    d. Increased socialization

20. Which of the following statements is true of older adults?

    a. The majority are in nursing homes.

    b. There is no decline in IQ with advancing age.

    c. Most older adults suffer from debilitating illnesses.

    d. There are minimal visual changes associated with aging.

Chapter 18   The Older Client

1. By 2020 adults over age 65 are projected to make up what percentage of the total U.S. population?

   a. 5%

   b. 11%

   c. 16%

   d. 20%

2. Which of the following is the greatest problem in the homebound elderly?

   a. Malnutrition

   b. Falls

   c. Uncontrolled diabetes

   d. Loneliness

3. Most elderly are hard of hearing, forgetful, rigid, and grumpy.

   ❑ True

   ❑ False

4. An expectation of the older adult in this stage of growth and development is to accept one's life as it is. Which of the following actions would facilitate this goal?

   a. Encourage the use of reminiscence.

   b. Assess for body image changes.

   c. Instruct about the benefits of proper nutrition and exercise.

   d. Encourage socialization.

5. The hearing loss associated with old age is called

   a. presbycusis.

   b. presbyopia.

   c. presbycardia.

   d. otitis media.

6. Match the pathologic visual change experienced by the elderly in the left column with its description from the right column.

_____ macular degeneration   a. Opacity of the lens of the eye

_____ cataracts   b. Inability of the lens to accommodate for near vision

_____ glaucoma   c. Increased intraocular pressure

_____ presbyopia   d. Loss of central vision

7. Which of the following physiological changes, associated with aging, would support the need to teach a preoperative 78-year-old client deep breathing, coughing, and incentive spirometry exercises?

   a. Fewer functioning alveoli and decrease in the number of cilia

   b. Decrease in peristaltic activity

   c. Slowed transmission of nerve impulses

   d. The development of lentigo senilis

8. The composition of body water to total body weight in an older adult is 40%.

   ❑ True

   ❑ False

9. Aging is associated with altered functioning of the pancreas. Which of the following would a nurse evaluate in order to assess this problem?

   a. Blood glucose level

   b. Blood urea nitrogen level

   c. Bowel sounds

   d. Blood potassium level

10. Mr. Palmer, 75 years old, states that his ejaculations are less forceful and he has to get up during the night several times to urinate. Are these symptoms associated with the normal aging process?

   ❑ Yes

   ❑ No

11. Kyphosis and osteoporosis in older women are most likely the result of *inactivity*.

   ❑ True

   ❑ False

12. Which of the following statements is true regarding wound healing in the elderly? Wounds heal

    a. at the same rate as in middle-aged adults.

    b. faster than in middle-aged adults.

    c. slower than in middle-aged adults.

13. Which of the following strategies would be appropriate to teach an elderly client regarding skin care?

    a. Avoid tub baths.

    b. Use tepid water during baths.

    c. Rub the skin briskly while drying the skin.

    d. Use alcohol to soothe itchy dry skin areas.

14. Mrs. Carpenter, 82 years old, was admitted to your unit yesterday with pneumonia. She is running a consistent low-grade fever, is dehydrated, and has difficulty getting out of bed due to stiffness in her right hip and knee joints. Her mental examination results in the following findings: she is disoriented, with the disorientation worsening at night; she mumbles incoherently at times; she has difficulty concentrating on simple tasks such as feeding herself; and she calls out in fear to the nurses to remove the bugs that are crawling up the privacy curtain in her room. Her son states that she was not this way at home, that she was alert and oriented. Which of the following best summarizes the clinical features of Mrs. Carpenter's mental status? She is

    a. acutely confused.

    b. suffering from dementia.

    c. experiencing an episode of depression.

    d. suffering from a personality disorder.

15. Polypharmacy places the elderly at risk for adverse drug reactions.

    ❑ True

    ❑ False

16. Match the age-related change in the left column with its impact on drug therapy from the right column.

_____ less total body fluid

_____ increased adipose tissue

_____ reduced liver size and decreased hepatic metabolism

_____ reduction in glomerular filtration rate, decrease in number of nephrons

_____ drier oral mucosa

_____ less muscle mass

_____ reduced circulation to lower bowel and vagina

a. Difficulty absorbing usual intramuscular adult dose at a single injection site

b. Higher level of water-soluble drugs

c. Greater accumulation of fat-soluble drugs

d. Slower metabolism and longer half-life of some drugs

e. Prolonged melting times for suppositories

f. Difficulty swallowing tablets and capsules

g. Slower elimination of some drugs

17. When taking a medication history of an elderly client, which of the following should be assessed in addition to the client's prescription drugs?

a. Potential interactions with foods

b. Use of over-the-counter medications

c. How medications are obtained

d. All of the above

18. Which of the following types of elder abuse is imposed social isolation?

a. Psychological abuse

b. Physical abuse

c. Neglect

d. Exploitation

19. List three age-related factors that contribute to falls.

1. _____

2. _____

3. _____

20. Mrs. Freidman was admitted to your long-term care facility today. Which of the following interventions would promote her safety during her stay?

a. Teach her about correct medication administration.

b. Orient her to her surroundings.

c. Provide large-print materials for her to read.

d. Help her to focus on her abilities instead of her limitations.

Chapter 19   Self-concept

1. Match the term in the left column with its definition from the right column.

   _____ identity   a. What an individual thinks he or she looks like

   _____ body image   b. Set of expected behaviors determined by family, culture, and society

   _____ role   c. A person's sense of self-worth

   _____ self-esteem   d. The set of characteristics a person is recognized by

2. Within which of the following life stages does the self-concept develop and change?

   a. Childhood

   b. Adolescence

   c. Adulthood

   d. All of the above

3. A client with a diagnosis of cancer is at risk for experiencing self-concept disturbance.

   ❑ True

   ❑ False

4. A nurse has school, family, and work demands and is having difficulty prioritizing which tasks to do first. Which of the following types of role conflict does this situation describe?

   a. Interrole conflict

   b. Interpersonal role conflict

   c. Role overload

   d. Person-role conflict

5. A nurse asks a client the following question during an interview: "What are your strengths and weaknesses?" Which of the following aspects of the self-concept does this question assess?

   a. Body image

   b. Identity

   c. Role

   d. Self-esteem

6. A client who presents with an external locus of control has high self-esteem.

   ❏ True

   ❏ False

7. Mr. Howard, a 59-year-old patient, was admitted to your unit for a lower GI bleed two days ago. He experienced incontinence of bloody stool on his first day of hospitalization. His PMH is unremarkable; this is his first hospital admission since a car accident when he was 20 years old. He is restless and becomes belligerent with the nursing staff when he is interrupted while on the telephone conducting office business. As you give him his medication he says, "I don't need these medicines; there is nothing wrong with me." Which of the following nursing diagnoses would be appropriate for Mr. Howard?

   a. Alteration in defense mechanisms

   b. Self-concept disturbance

   c. Hopelessness

   d. Social isolation

8. A 16-year-old female has been admitted for anorexia. When you collect the supper tray you notice that she has not eaten anything. When speaking to her about this, she says, "I can't eat; I am too fat already." Which of the following nursing diagnoses would most likely apply?

   a. Situational low self-esteem

   b. Anxiety

   c. Body image disturbance

   d. Self-esteem disturbance

9. Which of the following nursing interventions is directed at minimizing stress associated with illness?

   a. Verbally instructing the client's spouse about effects and side effects of medications

   b. Allowing the client decision making about timing of care activities

   c. Directing the client to ask the physician about postoperative care during hospitalization

   d. Asking the client how he or she has coped with past illnesses

10. The menopausal woman has decreased sex drive.

    ❑ True

    ❑ False

11. Which of the following goals would be appropriate for a client experiencing *situational low self-esteem?*

    a. The client will experience self-esteem.

    b. The client will state his positive attributes.

    c. The nurse will support the client's weaknesses.

    d. The nurse will facilitate the client's growth.

12. Recovery from illness is compromised when a client's anxiety level is high.

    ❑ True

    ❑ False

13. You notice your colleague: she is well-groomed, her posture is erect, her speech is articulate, she is able to maintain relationships appropriately, is self directed, and is able to take care of herself. Would you say that she has high or low self-esteem?

    ❑ High self-esteem

    ❑ Low self-esteem

14. In which of the following life stages would an individual's self-concept be most influenced by feedback from significant others?

    a. Childhood

    b. Adolescence

    c. Adulthood

    d. All of the above

15. Which of the following statements is true about self-concept?

    a. Self-concept is an individual's perception of self.

    b. Self-concept is the perception of others about an individual.

    c. Self-concept is the reflection of an individual's achievements.

    d. Self-concept is derived from the expectations of others for an individual.

Chapter 20   Stress, Anxiety, and Adaptation

1. Match the term in the left column with its definition from the right column.

    _____ stress

    _____ stressor

    _____ anxiety

    _____ adaptation

    _____ homeostasis

    _____ maladaptation

    _____ eustress

    _____ distress

    a. The body's reaction to any stimulus

    b. The ineffective response to stressors

    c. Any situation, event, or agent that threatens a person's security

    d. The process whereby a person adjusts to stressors

    e. Ineffective coping with stressors

    f. The type of stress that results in positive outcomes

    g. A subjective response to a threat to a person's well-being

    h. A steady state balancing physiological, psychological, sociocultural, intellectual, and spiritual needs

2. Which of the following types of stressors is a hot, crowded, noisy subway?

    a. Physiological

    b. Psychological

    c. Environmental

    d. Sociocultural

3. When the autonomic nervous system is aroused, the sympathetic nervous system response results in a *decrease* in heart rate.

    ❏ True

    ❏ False

4. Which of the following is a cognitive manifestation of stress?

    a. Impaired judgment

    b. Headache

    c. Insomnia

    d. Social isolation

5. When a client is in a situational crisis, this client is considered temporarily mentally ill.

    ❑ True

    ❑ False

6. Mr. Orapollo, during a routine visit for his diabetes management, states that he is having trouble sleeping, difficulty concentrating, "flies off the handle" at his wife, and cannot find any interest to sufficiently occupy his time since his retirement a month ago. Which of the following type of crisis is Mr. Orapollo most likely in?

    a. Maturational

    b. Situational

    c. Adventitious

    d. Diabetic

7. Which of the following is an appropriate nursing intervention for a client whose anxiety level is severe?

    a. Discuss medication side effects and dosing instructions.

    b. Assist the client in linking the stressor to the anxiety response.

    c. Invite the client to join a group on diet management.

    d. Using broad opening statements, allow the client an opportunity to discuss concerns.

8. The theorist who proposed that the change process occurs in the three stages of unfreezing, moving, and refreezing is

    a. Freud.

    b. Lippitt.

    c. Lewin.

    d. Nelson.

9. Match the defense mechanism in the left column with an example of it from the right column.

_____ denial
a. A nurse comes to work after an argument with her husband and becomes angry with the nurse's aide.

_____ displacement
b. A workaholic mother brings a gift home every day to her child.

_____ rationalization
c. A client blames his wife for misplacing items when he cannot remember where he put things.

_____ regression
d. A student nurse puts his children out of his mind while he is studying for an examination.

_____ suppression
e. A client says he can't follow the prescribed diet because his wife doesn't know how to cook the proper foods.

_____ repression
f. A client with cirrhosis continues to heavily drink alcohol.

_____ projection
g. A 54-year-old patient with bone cancer refuses to feed himself during hospitalization.

_____ reaction formation
h. A client is unaware of her sexual abuse history.

10. When a client benefits from the sick role by gaining attention and sympathy, this is called a _____ _____.

11. There is a relationship between stress experienced by a client and immune system function.
❑ True
❑ False

12. Ms. Marrow has come to the emergency room with a fractured right arm. She states she fell down the stairs at home. The hospital records indicate Ms. Marrow has been to the emergency room twice in the past six months for a head concussion and a miscarriage. As you interview Ms. Marrow, you learn she has experienced several losses recently, one of which was the death of her mother. She appears shy and scared. You learn that she is taking antidepressants for "the blues I can't shake." When you ask her how the fall happened, she states, "These things just keep happening to me. I can't stop them." Which of the following nursing diagnoses would be appropriate for Ms. Marrow?

a. Ineffective denial

b. Powerlessness

c. Ineffective coping

d. Depression

13. Which of the following phrases explains the benefits of catharsis as a therapeutic intervention for purposes of anxiety management?

   a. Once a feeling is described, it is real and can be dealt with.

   b. It reduces the tension in muscles.

   c. It clarifies the message of the sender for the receiver.

   d. It allows the nurse to offer an opinion on the client's experience.

14. One of the beneficial effects of exercise in managing stress is the stimulation of the production of endorphins. Which of the following best describes endorphins? Endorphins are

   a. a group of naturally occurring, chemically related, long-chain hydroxy fatty acids that stimulate the contractility of smooth muscles.

   b. a group of opiate-like substances produced naturally by the brain that raise the body's pain threshold.

   c. a group of high-molecular-weight kininogens that increase the permeability of capillaries.

   d. intermediate products in the synthesis of norepinephrine, a neurotransmitter.

15. Your client is having difficulty falling asleep. Which of the following stress management strategies would you recommend?

   a. Progressive muscle relaxation

   b. Exercise

   c. Guided imagery

   d. Aromatherapy

16. Match the stress management technique in the left column with its definition from the right column.

_____	biofeedback	a. Noise, sound, light, and other stimuli in the client's immediate surroundings are manipulated.
_____	progressive muscle relaxation	b. Clients learn to manipulate body responses through mental activity.
_____	guided imagery	c. The client tenses and releases muscle groups throughout the body, paying attention to sensations of tension and relaxation.
_____	cognitive reframing	d. The client's perception and interpretations are altered by changing of the client's thoughts.
_____	environmental strategies	e. A client is guided through a pleasant scene, using all the senses, in order to become fully relaxed.

17. Which of the following assessments would not be useful when evaluating the effectiveness of anxiety reduction strategies?

    a. Vital signs measurement

    b. Cognition

    c. Motor movement

    d. Oxygen saturation

18. Would you recommend the avoidance of alcohol, tobacco, and caffeine to an overstressed colleague as part of a stress management plan?

    ❏ Yes

    ❏ No

19. The first step in managing the stress leading to burnout is to change work environments.

    ❏ True

    ❏ False

20. Which of the following hormones is *not* involved in the biological changes associated with the fight-or-flight responses?

    a. Adrenalin

    b. Thyroid hormone

    c. Norepinephrine

    d. Glucocorticoids

Chapter 21 Loss and Grief

1. Match the term in the left column with its definition from the right column.

   _____ actual loss   a. Loss of a body part or body function

   _____ perceived loss   b. Loss of an aspect of self that is not physical; for example, loss of humor

   _____ physical loss   c. The period of grief following the death of a loved one

   _____ psychological loss   d. An adaptive process related to loss

   _____ grief   e. A series of intense physical and psychological responses that occur following a loss

   _____ mourning   f. Loss felt by an individual but not tangible to others

   _____ bereavement   g. Death of a loved one; theft of an object

2. A middle-aged woman experiencing menopause is an example of *situational* loss.

   ❑ True

   ❑ False

3. Mrs. Yankovsky, age 30, is two days post-op for the removal of her uterus and ovaries as a result of uterine and ovarian cancer. The cancer has metastasized to other body areas. Her husband is troubled by his wife's illness; she had previously been healthy. He wanted to have more children. He acts very anxious when the nurses enter the room to give care. Which of the following statements best describes the losses this couple is facing?

   a. Loss of good health, goals, bodily function, and self-concept as a whole

   b. Loss of role relationship, body parts, hope, and job

   c. Loss of a significant other, self-concept, body parts, and support

4. Which of the following theorists stated, "Grief results when an individual experiences a disruption in attachment to a love object"?

   a. Bowlby

   b. Worden

   c. Engle

   d. Lindemann

5. Which of the following phrases best describes a person who has experienced a loss and subsequently does not experience the emotions associated with grief or does not demonstrate the typical behaviors associated with grief?

   a. Uncomplicated grief

   b. Dysfunctional grief

   c. Anticipatory grief

   d. Normal grief

6. Which of the following stages of mourning, according to Engle, would a person who experienced a loss be in for 6–12 months? During this time, the person is experiencing feelings of sadness, isolation, and loneliness.

   a. Stage I

   b. Stage II

   c. Stage III

7. The cause of death affects the intensity and duration of the grief response.

   ❏ True

   ❏ False

8. Which of the following nursing interventions is appropriate for a 4-year-old child who has recently experienced the death of a parent?

   a. Take the child to the cemetery.

   b. Reassure the child that the child did not contribute to the cause of death.

   c. Tell the child that the fear of death is irrational.

   d. Tell the child the parent is in "a kind of sleep."

9. Mrs. Crowley is hospitalized and dying of bowel cancer. Her husband approaches you angrily, saying that his wife is receiving substandard care. Which of the following responses would be most helpful?

   a. "I understand that you want the best for your wife. Tell me what it is that is bothering you about her care."

   b. "I know it is difficult for both you and your wife, but we are doing the best we can."

   c. "I apologize. We have been understaffed for the past two days."

   d. "I will contact the charge nurse and we will discuss this matter."

10. Matthew, age 6, is dying. He has been suffering with leukemia for three years and is no longer responding to treatment. His mother has difficulty sleeping and eating and feels guilty for not "quitting smoking" while she was pregnant with Matthew. She blames herself for his illness. Which of the following nursing diagnoses is most appropriate for Matthew's mother?

   a. Grieving

   b. Anticipatory grieving

   c. Dysfunctional grieving

   d. Distorted grief

11. Match the Kübler-Ross stage of death and dying in the left column with an example of a client's statement or behavior from the right column that best exemplifies the stage.

   _____ denial   a. The client arranges his own wake and funeral.

   _____ anger   b. The client wants to be left alone.

   _____ bargaining   c. A client states, "Doctor, I want to live long enough to see my daughter get married."

   _____ depression   d. A client diagnosed with heart failure continues to eat foods high in sodium and cholesterol.

   _____ acceptance   e. A client states, "You don't know anything about taking care of someone like me."

12. Depression experienced as part of the dying process assists a client to detach from life.
   ❑ True
   ❑ False

13. Which of the following would be most important to know in order to plan for the care of a dying client?

   a. The availability of a support system

   b. The client's oxygenation status

   c. The client's hydration status

   d. The availability of hospice care

14. Which of the following in Maslow's Hierarchy of Needs is a priority when caring for a dying client?

   a. Physiological needs

   b. Self-esteem needs

   c. Self-actualization needs

   d. Love and belonging needs

15. A regular around-the-clock (ATC) administration of analgesics surpasses the therapeutic effectiveness of PRN administration of analgesics.

    ❑ True

    ❑ False

16. Match the physiological change after death in the left column with the nursing care implication in the right column.

    _____ algor mortis   a. The head should be elevated.

    _____ liver mortis   b. Carefully remove tape and dressing materials from the body.

    _____ rigor mortis   c. Dentures should be inserted, the eyes closed, and the body positioned soon after death.

17. Which of the following is the greatest fear of dying clients?

    a. Loss of independence

    b. Loss of mobility

    c. Pain

    d. Dying alone

18. An autopsy is necessary in the case of a client on a medical-surgical unit who dies of cancer two weeks after admission.

    ❑ True

    ❑ False

19. Would you agree or disagree that the following statement is an indicator of successful grieving? A client remembers the deceased in an idealized manner.

    ❑ Agree

    ❑ Disagree

20. Euthanasia is considered ethical practice in the profession of nursing.

    ❑ True

    ❑ False

Chapter 22 Professional Accountability and Leadership

1. While you are waiting for class to begin, you overhear two of your colleagues discussing nursing as a profession.

   Nursing student A: "Nursing *is* a true profession; it has a professional organization, the American Nurses Association, and nurses are required to be licensed in order to practice."

   Nursing student B: "Since the beginning of the 20th century, nursing has attempted to meet the criteria of a profession."

   Which of these nursing students' statements most accurately reflects the state of nursing as a profession?

   a. Nursing student A

   b. Nursing student B

2. As a practicing nurse in a coronary care unit, you join the American Association of Critical Care Nurses. Does your action support nursing in its attempt to be a profession?

   ❏ Yes

   ❏ No

3. To which of the following groups is a nurse accountable?

   a. The client and the client's family

   b. The nursing profession

   c. The employer

   d. All of the above

4. Match the term in the left column with its definition from the right column.

    _____ professional regulation   a. The law governing nursing practice within a state

    _____ professional standards   b. Process by which a nongovernmental agency states that an individual licensed to practice a profession has met predetermined standards set for practice

    _____ accreditation   c. The method by which states hold the individual nurse accountable for safe practice to citizens of that state

    _____ certification   d. Process by which nursing ensures that its members act in the public interest

    _____ scope of practice   e. Statements by which quality of service, practice, and education can be judged

    _____ nurse practice act   f. Legal boundaries of practice set by state statutes

    _____ licensure   g. An agency granting status to an institution that has met predetermined criteria

5. A nurse who takes a position in the emergency room of a busy metropolitan hospital registers for an Advanced Cardiac Life Support (ACLS) course. This action demonstrates professional accountability.

    ❑ True

    ❑ False

6. A candidate for licensure by endorsement is required to retake the NCLEX-RN.

    ❑ True

    ❑ False

7. Which of the following best explains the impetus for establishing the mutual recognition model for nurse licensure?

    a. The increase in the number of nurses who hold licensure in more than one state

    b. The increase in practice occurring across state lines.

8. Which of the following organizations prepares students to become contributing members of the nursing profession?

    a. NSNA (National Student Nurses Association)

    b. ANA (American Nurses Association)

    c. NLN (National League for Nursing)

    d. ICN (International Council of Nurses)

9. Which of the following organizations promotes nursing accountability by establishing educational standards and surveying schools of nursing?

   a. ANA

   b. ICN

   c. JCAHO

   d. NLN

10. State and federal agencies can access actions taken against professional nursing licensees from a data bank.

    ❑ True

    ❑ False

11. List three methods the nursing profession uses to ensure accountability to the public.

    1. _____

    2. _____

    3. _____

12. By which of the following methods does a State Board of Nursing hold an individual accountable for safe practice?

    a. Ensuring that individuals adhere to the nursing code of ethics

    b. Developing national standards of nursing practice

    c. Requiring individuals to pass an examination that determines the minimum level of practice competency

    d. Working with JCAHO to establish standards for safe practice and monitoring for any breach of safe practice

13. Match the type of leadership style in the left column with an example of it from the right column.

    _____ autocratic

    _____ democratic

    _____ laissez-faire

    _____ situational

    a. The unit manager allows an aggressive staff member to consistently dominate the staff meetings.

    b. The leader of the risk management committee is directive at times, while at other times lets the group problem-solve.

    c. The case manager gives background information about the client's case to the multidisciplinary team, and then invites discussion about the client's plan of care.

    d. The unit manager tells the staff what will be done to solve the unit's staffing problem.

14. In which of the following styles of leadership would the expected outcome be the empowerment of group members?

    a. Autocratic

    b. Democratic

    c. Laissez-faire

15. The UAP assigned to your unit approaches you and asks if she can change the dressing around your patient's G-tube. Which of the following questions would you *first* answer in order to make a decision whether to delegate this task to the UAP?

    a. Is the person competent to do the task?

    b. Can this task be delegated?

    c. If I delegate this task, will it put my patient at risk?

    d. What do the physician's orders say about this?

16. Does the way one dress influence the power dynamics in an interpersonal situation?

    ❑ Yes

    ❑ No

17. Sharing information with colleagues empowers everyone.

    ❑ True

    ❑ False

18. Which of the following reflects positive mentor behavior?

    a. An experienced staff nurse readily offers the answer to any questions.

    b. A unit manager allows a novice nurse to find a solution to a clinical problem.

    c. The chairperson of a newly formed committee allows the committee members to find their own direction.

    d. A nursing instructor offers to coach a nursing student in exchange for babysitting services.

19. You are the only nurse on your unit who knows how to use a special device that places pressure on a blood vessel after cardiac catheterization (Femstop). Which of the following types of power do you hold?

    a. Legitimate

    b. Referent

    c. Expert

    d. Reward

20. List three networking strategies you can use to increase your power base with colleagues.

1. _____

2. _____

3. _____

Chapter 23 Legal Accountability and Responsibilities

1. Which of the following mandates is the result of state administrative law action?

    a. Controlled Substances Act

    b. Nurse Practice Act

    c. Social Security Act

    d. National Labor Relations Act

2. Match the term in the left column with its definition in the right column.

    _____ malpractice   a. Person being sued

    _____ negligence   b. Breach of duty

    _____ plaintiff   c. Wrongful conduct by a professional

    _____ defendant   d. Party seeking damages

    _____ testimony   e. Written or verbal evidence given by an expert in an area

3. Place the following elements for the proof of liability in the proper sequence.

    _____ Injury is established.

    _____ There was an obligation created by law, contract, or any voluntary action.

    _____ A cause and effect is established linking the breach of duty to the injury.

    _____ An act of omission or commission caused a breach of duty.

4. Under which of the following conditions is it legal to apply restraints?

    a. When a client is confused

    b. When a client is in danger of harming himself or harming others

    c. When a client is agitated

    d. When a client is threatening to leave the hospital against medical advice (AMA)

5. Which of the following actions by a nurse demonstrates an understanding of a patient's right to privacy? The nurse

    a. checks on the patient using the intercom.

    b. ensures the noise level in a patient's room is kept to a minimum.

    c. knocks before entering a room.

    d. limits the visitors of a seriously ill patient.

6. A nurse is overheard in the elevator discussing a neighbor, saying he was recently diagnosed with AIDS. This nurse can be held liable for

    a. slander.

    b. libel.

    c. fraud.

7. Persons with psychiatric disorders are covered by the Americans with Disabilities Act (ADA).

    ❏ True

    ❏ False

8. To what standard would a nurse be held to when responding to an emergency in the community?

    a. By how a reasonable and prudent caregiver would have acted in the same situation.

    b. The nurse has full immunity from litigation.

    c. By the standards set forth in the local community hospital for emergency care.

    d. The nurse has full immunity as long as no money is accepted for the care rendered during the emergency.

9. A client refuses her Vitamin K injection. The nurse administers it against the client's will. Can this nurse be found guilty of assault and battery?

    ❏ Yes

    ❏ No

10. You notice that a coworker's patient has received three doses of narcotic analgesics throughout your shift, as documented on the MAR; however, the patient continues to complain of pain. You remember that two days ago a similar occurrence happened when you worked with this colleague. You suspect that this person is signing out narcotic analgesics, documenting the analgesics were given, but not administering the analgesics to the patient. What should you do?

    a. Nothing

    b. Monitor the situation

    c. Report this coworker to the nursing supervisor

    d. Report this coworker to the State Board of Nursing

11. Nurses who are covered by their employer's liability insurance do not need to purchase their own individual liability insurance policy.

    ❑ True

    ❑ False

12. List four areas in nursing practice where nurses are at legal risk.

    1. _____

    2. _____

    3. _____

    4. _____

13. A nurse who does not belong to a union must float when reassigned to another unit.

    ❑ True

    ❑ False

14. A client falls and injures herself while under your care. Which of the following actions would you take to decrease the risk of liability to you?

    a. Document the incident carefully on an incident report form.

    b. Chart the facts surrounding the client's fall, client condition, and follow-up care.

    c. Do not document anything about the fall.

    d. Remove yourself as a caregiver for this client.

15. Is a nurse legally liable for incorrectly administering a medication even if it was ordered incorrectly by a physician?

    ❑ Yes

    ❑ No

16. The role of the nurse in obtaining an informed consent for a surgical procedure is to witness the signature.

   ❑ True

   ❑ False

17. Does the law require the nurse to obtain formal informed consent prior to the initiation of nursing procedures?

   ❑ Yes

   ❑ No

18. In which of the following documents would a nurse seek to learn the name of the responsible person appointed by the client to make health care decisions for a client when the client is unable to make his or her health care decisions.

   a. Durable power of attorney

   b. Living will

   c. Advance care medical directive

   d. General consent form

19. Risk management programs are aimed at decreasing the risk of financial loss to the

   a. physician.

   b. agency.

   c. physician and nurse.

   d. agency, physician, and nurse.

20. Which of the following is the purpose of DNR physician's orders?

   a. To document the terminal nature of the patient's condition

   b. To allow an alternative to the universal standing order to provide cardiopulmonary resuscitation to all patients

   c. To provide an opportunity for the patient, family, and caregivers to discuss the nature of the patient's condition and the best possible course of action if the patient has a cardiac arrest

   d. To provide legal protection for nurses who believe a patient should not be resuscitated

Chapter 24 Ethical Obligations and Accountability

1. Match the term in the left column with its definition from the right column.

   _____ ethics

   _____ morals

   _____ values

   _____ ethical principles

   _____ bioethics

   a. The personal beliefs held by an individual that reflect religion or tradition

   b. What a person considers of worth, indirectly impacting behavior

   c. The application of ethical principles to health care

   d. Codes that direct or govern our actions

   e. The branch of philosophy that concerns the distinction of right and wrong on the basis of a body of knowledge

2. Deontology states that value of a situation is determined by its consequences.

   ❑ True

   ❑ False

3. The Nightengale Pledge states that while clients are under the care of a nurse, the nurse is to do no harm to the client. Which of the following ethical principles does this represent?

   a. Justice

   b. Nonmaleficence

   c. Fidelity

   d. Beneficence

4. Match the ethical principle in the left column with an appropriate example from the right column.

_____	autonomy	a.	The nurse represents the client's viewpoint accurately during the interdisciplinary conference.
_____	nonmaleficence	b.	A client is asked to sign an informed consent form by a physician.
_____	beneficence	c.	The nurse signs for a wasted narcotic only after she sees it being discarded.
_____	justice	d.	The nurse triple checks the medication for "right medication and right dose."
_____	veracity	e.	The nurse considers whether a client should be physically restrained.
_____	fidelity	f.	The client assignments on the unit are equally divided among the nurses.

5. The values of the nurse have little impact on the delivery of care.

❑ True

❑ False

6. List three frequently occurring ethical dilemmas in health care.

1. _____

2. _____

3. _____

7. The Board of Nursing has the authority to reprimand a nurse for unprofessional conduct for a violation of the American Nurses Association (ANA) Code of Ethics.

❑ True

❑ False

8. Which of the following is *not* included in the American Hospital Association (1972) "Patient's Bill of Rights"?

a. The patient has the right to considerate and respectful care.

b. The patient has the right to make decisions about the plan of care.

c. The patient has the right to have an advance directive concerning treatment.

d. The patient has the right to sign a release of responsibility and leave the hospital at any time.

9. Would you agree with the following statement? One of the obligations the nursing profession owes to society is for its practitioners to behave with high ethical standards.

   ❑ Yes

   ❑ No

10. A nurse is bound by the ANA Code of Ethics to preserve a client's right to privacy.

    ❑ True

    ❑ False

11. You are making an initial home care visit with Mrs. Lanscomb's nurse. Mrs. Lanscomb has recently been discharged from the hospital with a diagnosis of congestive heart failure and diabetes. After the assessment and interview, the nurse sits down with Mrs. Lanscomb and develops a plan of care to assist her in managing her medications and activities of daily living. Which of the following patient rights is the nurse preserving?

    a. The right to make decisions regarding her care

    b. Her right to be involved in the treatment process

    c. The right to be treated with dignity and respect

    d. All of the above

12. In which of the following steps in the ethical decision-making process would the ethical dilemma be stated?

    a. Determination of claims and identification of parties

    b. Problem identification

    c. Generation of alternatives

    d. Assessing the outcome of moral actions

13. Which of the following best defines an ethical dilemma?

    a. A conflict between two or more ethical principles

    b. A conflict between the interests of two or more parties in the care of an individual

    c. A choice between two equally satisfactory alternatives

    d. A choice between the desired action of the nurse and the client

14. Will there be a right or wrong decision after deliberating an ethical dilemma?

    ❑ Yes

    ❑ No

15. Match the term in the left column with its definition from the right column.

_____ euthanasia   a. Taking deliberate action that hastens a client's death

_____ active euthanasia   b. The omission of an action that would prolong a client's life

_____ passive euthanasia   c. A health care professional providing the client with the means to end his or her own life

_____ assisted suicide   d. The deliberate ending of a life as a human action

16. What is the ANA position on the participation of nurses in active euthanasia?

a. Participation is in violation of nursing's ethical code.

b. Participation is sanctioned only when the circumstances clearly warrant such action.

c. Nursing's ethical code stands in support of active euthanasia.

17. Nurses are fully protected from employer reprisal when they "blow the whistle" on incompetent coworkers.

❑ True

❑ False

18. Which of the following behaviors is unethical and illegal?

a. Taking narcotics from the narcotic cabinet for your own use

b. Assisting a physician in an abortion clinic to perform an abortion

c. Allowing a gay (homosexual) AIDS patient to sleep with his partner in the hospital

d. Giving out patient information over the telephone to a spouse

19. **Patient:** "What is this medication for?"

Nurse: "It regulates your heart beat."

Patient: "I don't think I want to take it; my heart is fine now."

Nurse: "Just take it. We know what's best for you."

Is the nurse's response considered paternalistic?

❑ Yes

❑ No

20. Mrs. Edwards is diagnosed with cancer of the bowel and is recovering from a bowel resection. Her husband comes to you and asks you not to tell her that she has cancer. He instructs you to make her believe that the surgery has relieved her bowel obstruction. His intent is to prevent her from unnecessary worry. Which of the following ethical principles are conflicting?

    a. Veracity and beneficence

    b. Veracity and nonmaleficence

    c. Justice and beneficence

    d. Fidelity and justice

Chapter 25   The Role of Quality Management in Accountability

1. Participation in JCAHO accreditation is required of all health care delivery provider organizations by the federal Health Care Finance Administration.

   ❑ True

   ❑ False

2. Match the terms on the left with the appropriate definition on the right.

   _____ quality assurance   a. Meeting or exceeding requirements of the customer

   _____ quality domains   b. Structure, process, and outcome

   _____ dimensions of quality performance   c. A method of management that views the employee as a resource

   _____ quality   d. Problem solving to work toward quality care

   _____ continuous quality improvement   e. The scientific approach used to study work processes

   _____ total quality management   f. Efficacy, appropriateness, availability, timeliness, effectiveness, continuity, safety, efficiency, respect, and caring

3. Medical errors are a significant cause of death and injury in the U.S. To minimize these occurrences, it is recommended that

   a. individuals be held accountable for these errors.

   b. work flow enhancements are put into place.

   c. system errors are corrected.

4. During a team meeting, the unit manager reports that the patients are increasingly complaining that their call lights are not being answered in a timely fashion. Staff nurse Smith says to her coworker, staff nurse Jennings, "There is nothing we can do about it. We are so short-staffed." Nurse Jennings, who knows that quality improvement is a team responsibility, says:

   a. "We could really use extra help, but it is up to the hospital administration to let us hire more staff."

   b. "I'm sure we can manage if we all pitch in."

   c. "We should all meet to study the problem together and develop some solutions."

   d. "Don't look at me, I answer my patients' call lights as soon as I can."

5. As of January 2000, JACHO discontinued the practice of conducting unannounced visits.

   ❑ True

   ❑ False

6. Which of the following terms best describes the method of management that was dominant during the mid-20th century?

   a. Controlling

   b. Collaboration

   c. Goal-setting

7. The _____ is accountable for performance improvement.

   a. facility director

   b. individual employee

   c. unit manager

   d. customer

8. Failure to adhere to federally mandated health care standards by health care facilities can result in which of the following actions?

   a. The chief operating officer can be arrested.

   b. Employees can be dismissed at will.

   c. Federal funding and payment can be denied.

   d. The facility can be shut down.

9. Which of the following federal regulations established denial of payment for substandard care?

   a. Consolidated Omnibus Budget Reconciliation Act

   b. Social Security Act

   c. Omnibus Budget Reconciliation Act

   d. Patient Self Determination Act

10. Total quality management (TQM) is a systems approach to quality management.

   ❑ True

   ❑ False

11. A staff nurse in a hospital is responsible for providing direct care to patients and considers a patient as a customer. To what other customers is the nurse accountable within the hospital?

_____

_____

_____

_____

12. Which of the following skills is essential to the TQM process?

a. Reporting problems in a timely fashion

b. Collating data from patient satisfaction surveys

c. Completing occurrence forms accurately

d. Listening to clients express their concerns about care

13. Which of the following organizational characteristics would you expect to find in a high performance organization?

a. The organization operates hierarchically.

b. Conflict is welcome, considered helpful.

c. The atmosphere is political.

d. The staff are the authority on care of the client.

14. List three characteristics of quality nursing care.

1. _____

2. _____

3. _____

15. In a unit meeting, the unit manager reported that the readmission rate of surgical patients had increased. The primary reason for readmission was wound infection. In this situation, which of the following health care providers carries the responsibility for quality improvement?

a. The nurses

b. The physicians

c. The unlicensed assistive personnel

d. All health care providers

16. Which term refers to the collection of data from client records and the subsequent comparison of this data to a set of predetermined criteria?

_____

17. Place the following steps of the scientific approach for improving quality performance in the order of their occurrence.

_____ Assess variations.

_____ Implement change in the process.

_____ Identify an important process to evaluate.

_____ Formulate improvements.

_____ Measure the current process.

18. As a nursing unit manager, you learn from the patient satisfaction surveys that patients are dissatisfied with the lengthy wait periods during transfers to and from the radiology department. You also learn that there are complaints about the lack of courtesy of the transport people and the radiology staff. Which of the following types of process improvement would you initiate?

    a. Cross-functional team

    b. Functional team

19. Sally, a coworker, comes to you and states that the hospital across the river has a shorter length of stay for the same surgery that is performed on the patients on your unit. She suggests that this information can be used as benchmarking data. Do you agree that this is an appropriate source of data for benchmarking purposes?

    ❑ Yes

    ❑ No

20. Health care will be delivered by a more diverse workforce in the 21st century. This phenomenon will affect the methods of delivery of health care.

    ❑ True

    ❑ False

Chapter 26   Accountability: Documentation and Reporting

1. The documentation of nursing care in the client record reflects the use of the nursing process.

   ❑ True

   ❑ False

2. JCAHO determines the type of document used by a health care organization.

   ❑ True

   ❑ False

3. Which of the following is the best defense of a nurse during a malpractice lawsuit?

   a. Depositions by fellow nurses

   b. The client record

   c. Character witnesses

   d. Personal anecdotal notes

4. Which of the following statements best describes the information contained in the consultation sheet found in the medical record?

   a. It contains medical orders and the treatment plan.

   b. It contains a record of the client's vital signs.

   c. It contains a record of the history and physical examination conducted by the attending physician.

   d. It contains a request for the services of other practitioners.

5. While reviewing a client record, you come upon a form that includes information about the client's wishes regarding life-sustaining procedures if the client becomes unable to make these decisions. This form is a(n)

   a. durable power of attorney for health care.

   b. advance directive.

   c. informed consent.

   d. incident form.

6. Which of the following statements best interprets the signature of an informed consent form by a nurse as witness to the client's signature?

   a. The client understands the procedure written on the consent form.

   b. The physician has explained the procedure to the client.

   c. The client is, in fact, the client and is competent to make a decision.

   d. The nurse was assigned to the client at the time of obtaining the informed consent.

7. JCAHO requires that health care organizations include nursing care plans in the client record.

   ❑ True

   ❑ False

8. Compliance with COBRA is monitored by the federal government by retrospective medical record review.

   ❑ True

   ❑ False

9. Which of the following statements depicts the correct action to take if you make a documentation mistake on the medical record?

   a. Erase the mistake and write over it.

   b. Scratch it out so it is completely obliterated.

   c. Cross it out and go on with the recording.

   d. Draw one line through it, and sign and date the correction.

10. Which of the following organizations approves abbreviations and symbols for use in a medical record?

    a. ANA

    b. AMA

    c. NANDA

    d. The health care organization

11. If you make a medication error, should this be documented in the nurses' notes?

    ❑ Yes

    ❑ No

12. Match the method of documentation in the left column with its example or definition from the right column.

_____ narrative charting

_____ problem-oriented medical record

_____ PIE charting

_____ focus charting

_____ charting by exception

_____ computerized documentation

a. SOAP note entries are made in the medical record

b. Saves documentation time, increases legibility, and facilitates the statistical analysis of data

c. Flow sheets are used extensively; deviations from preestablished norms are documented

d. Uses a chronological, storytelling format

e. Charting uses a columnar format within the progress notes to distinguish it from other recordings in the narrative notes

f. Incorporates the ongoing plan of care into the daily charting

13. You accompany a home care nurse making a home visit. After leaving the home the nurse enters client data into a handheld computer. Which of the following best describes this documentation system? It is

    a. point-of-care charting.

    b. focus charting.

    c. narrative charting.

    d. none of the above.

14. Flow sheets eliminate the need for nurses' notes.

    ❑ True

    ❑ False

15. Which of the following nurses' note entries in the medical record is most accurate?

    a. Pt. is able to deep breathe and cough without difficulty.

    b. Pt. performs deep breathing and coughing exercises independently; cough is nonproductive.

    c. Pt. assisted with deep breathing and coughing (DB&C) exercising, expectorating small amounts of clear sputum. Lung sounds clear after DB&C activity.

    d. Pt. states deep breathing and coughing exercises are painful.

16. The Nursing Intervention Classification system labels nursing actions as interventions and includes them in the classification.

   ❑ True

   ❑ False

17. Which of the following is a necessary element in order for computerized documentation systems in health care agencies to demonstrate the quality, effectiveness, and value of nursing service?

   a. A standardized nursing language

   b. Standardized databases

   c. A final version of the nursing taxonomy

   d. Nurses who are able to improve patient care delivery systems

18. Which of the following is the most accurate entry on the physician's order sheet by a nurse after taking a telephone order from a physician?

   a. Give Lasix 40 mg IVP now
      T.O. Dr. Donohue/ Mary Smith R.N.

   b. Verapamil 5mg IVP stat
      Dr. Jones/ Mary Smith R.N.

   c. Dulcolax tablets for constipation
      Dr. Cordovan/ Mary Smith R.N.

   d. Tylenol 650 mg q 4–6h PRN for headache
      Mary Smith R.N.

19. It is recommended that nurses document a client incident of a fall carefully on the client record. Which of the following is the correct rationale for this?

   a. Falls are costly to treat.

   b. Falls are the main reason nurses are sued.

   c. The data is used by risk managers to identify factors that create risk for falls in a client population in a facility.

   d. The documentation assists the physician with diagnosing and treating the client's condition after the fall.

20. Which of the following documentation systems would the nurse be expected to use to document a variance from an expected outcome?

   a. Narrative charting

   b. Charting by exception

   c. Critical pathway

   d. Nursing care Kardex

Chapter 27 Vital Signs and Physical Assessment

1. *Internal respiration* is the exchange of oxygen and carbon dioxide between alveoli of the lungs and the pulmonary blood system.

   ❑ True

   ❑ False

2. Match the term in the left column with its definition from the right column.

   _____ hemodynamic regulation

   _____ systole

   _____ diastole

   _____ stroke volume

   _____ cardiac output

   _____ pulse pressure

   _____ blood pressure

   a. The phase in which the ventricles contract to eject blood

   b. The measurement of pressure pulsations exerted against the blood vessel walls during systole and diastole

   c. The maintenance of an appropriate environment in tissue fluids

   d. The measurement of blood that enters the aorta with each ventricular contraction

   e. The volume of blood pumped in one minute

   f. The phase in which ventricles are relaxed and no blood is being ejected

   g. The measurement of the ratio of stroke volume to compliance of the arterial system

3. You assess the pulse of a 1-year-old infant. The normal range of pulse for this infant is

   a. 60–80 bpm.

   b. 80–110 bpm.

   c. 80–170 bpm.

   d. 100–200 bpm.

4. Before you take Mr. Seaforth's vital signs, you ask him what medications he is taking. He responds by saying that he is taking digitalis once a day in the morning. Which of the following vital sign changes would you expect to find when assessing his vital signs?

   a. Increased blood pressure

   b. Decreased pulse rate

   c. Decreased respiratory rate

   d. Increased temperature

5. An increased anxiety level causes an increase in the heart rate and a decrease in the blood pressure.

   ❑ True

   ❑ False

6. You are teaching Mr. Cain to monitor his fluid retention by weighing himself every day. Which of the following instructions would be appropriate during this teaching episode?

   a. Weigh yourself at the same time each day wearing the same type of clothing.

   b. Make sure you eat first before you weigh yourself.

   c. The time of day is not important; however, make sure you wear the same type of clothing each day.

7. Which of the following routes of temperature measurement is least accurate?

   a. Axillary

   b. Oral

   c. Tympanic

   d. Rectal

8. Which of the following techniques is appropriate to use when measuring an adult temperature using a tympanic thermometer? Before inserting the probe,

   a. pull the pinna upward and back.

   b. pull the pinna down and back.

   c. pull the pinna down and forward.

   d. pull the pinna upward and forward.

9. When environmental conditions produce an elevation in body temperature, diaphoresis results. This is an attempt to cool the body by which of the following methods of heat loss?

   a. Evaporation

   b. Convection

   c. Conduction

   d. Radiation

10. Which of the following methods is the proper technique to determine if a client is experiencing a pulse deficit?

    a. Simultaneously have one person count the apical pulse and another person count the radial pulse.

    b. Measure the apical pulse, wait 20–30 minutes, and remeasure the apical pulse rate.

    c. Measure the radial pulse in each arm and subtract the difference.

    d. Measure the distal pulse with a pulse oximeter and compare this to the apical heart rate.

11. The proper placement of the stethoscope diaphragm while auscultating an apical pulse is at the 5th intercostal space on the left side of the anterior chest wall.

    ❑ True

    ❑ False

12. Match the term in the left column with its definition from the right column.

    _____ eupnea   a. Shallow respirations

    _____ bradypnea   b. Easy respirations of a normal rate

    _____ hypoventilation   c. Deep rapid respirations

    _____ tacypnea   d. A respiratory rate of 10 or lower

    _____ hyperventilation   e. Thoracic breathing

    _____ diaphragmatic breathing   f. A respiratory rate of 24 or above

    _____ costal breathing   g. Breathing from the abdomen

    _____ dyspnea   h. Labored or forceful breathing, using accessory muscles in the chest and neck

13. You enter Mr. Claus's room, introduce yourself, and explain that you will be measuring his vital signs. You note that in his left arm he has an IV infusing in the antecubital space and in his right hand there is a saline well (intermittent venous access device). In which arm would you measure Mr. Claus's blood pressure?

    a. Left arm

    b. Right arm

14. You are not confident with the first blood pressure measurement. How long should you wait before taking the second measurement?

    a. 30 seconds

    b. 1 minute

    c. 2 minutes

    d. 3 minutes

15. When a client has 20/40 vision it means that the client can read at a distance of 20 feet what a person with normal vision can read at a distance of 40 feet.

    ❑ True

    ❑ False

16. As you review a client's record, you read the notation "PERRLA." Which of the following organs does this notation pertain to?

    a. Eyes

    b. Ears

    c. Mouth

    d. Lungs

17. Match the term associated with respiratory assessment in the left column with its definition from the right column.

_____ aortic aneurysm

a. Heard over predominantly the base of the lungs as a fine, high-pitched popping sound of short duration

_____ atelectasis

b. High-pitched musical sounds that can be heard over all the lung fields

_____ bronchiectasis

c. A crowing sound heard predominantly on inspiration

_____ empyema

d. Accumulation of fluid in the interstitial and air spaces of the lung

_____ pleural effusion

e. Accumulation of pus in the pleural cavity

_____ stridor

f. Dilation and destruction of the bronchial walls

_____ pleural friction rub

g. Localized dilation of the aortic wall

_____ wheezes

h. Collapse of lung tissue and decreased gas exchange

_____ rhonchi

i. Heard predominantly on expiration over the trachea and bronchi as a low-pitched musical sound

_____ crackles

j. Heard as a continuous creaking, grating sound over the anterior chest wall

18. The heart sound S_3 is a normal heart sound.

❑ True

❑ False

19. You read on your client's medical record that the client has a Grade II heart murmur. Which of the following is most likely the cause of this finding?

a. Mitral regurgitation

b. A bundle branch block

c. Pneumothorax

d. Angina

20. In report you hear that your patient has hypoactive bowel sounds. Which of the following is the appropriate length of time you would listen to accurately assess bowel sounds?

a. 15 seconds in each quadrant

b. 30 seconds in each quadrant

c. 45 seconds in each quadrant

d. 1 minute in each quadrant

21. You are the intake coordinator at a home care agency. The transfer summary of your new client reads, under "Integumentary Assessment," that she has petechia on her arms and legs. How would you expect your patient's arms and legs to appear upon assessment? The extremities would appear to have

    a. purplish blue lesions with fading areas of green and yellow.

    b. flat, round 1–3 mm lesions that are reddish purple.

    c. spiderlike lesions of varying size and bluish in color.

22. Which of the following assessments would provide information about cerebellar function?

    a. Level of consciousness assessment data

    b. Assessment data regarding cranial nerve function

    c. Assessment of muscle tone and strength

    d. Assessment of the client's gait

23. How many kilograms does a 165-pound man weigh?

    a. 363 kg

    b. 7.5 kg

    c. 36.3 kg

    d. 75 kg

24. What is the minimum length of time to wait before measuring the oral temperature of a client who has taken a drink of ice water?

    a. No wait is necessary

    b. 5 minutes

    c. 15 minutes

    d. 45 minutes

25. A bulging of the anterior vaginal wall due to the protrusion of the urinary bladder indicates a _____.

Chapter **28** *Diagnostic Testing*

1. Prolonged application of a tourniquet can produce hemoconcentration in a blood sample.

   ❑ True

   ❑ False

2. When a tourniquet is properly applied for the purpose of venipuncture, both the venous and arterial blood flow is obstructed.

   ❑ True

   ❑ False

3. Which of the following methods is considered most reliable when identifying a client prior to a diagnostic procedure?

   a. Asking the client to state his or her name

   b. Checking the arm or leg band

   c. Asking a family member the client's name

   d. Checking the chart that accompanies the client

4. You are preparing your patient for a thoracentesis. Would you expect that the physician will order an analgesic or sedative as part of the preprocedure orders?

   ❑ Yes

   ❑ No

5. The result of the Allen test performed on your client's extremity is negative. Should an arterial puncture be performed on this extremity?

   ❑ Yes

   ❑ No

6. A urine specimen for culture is obtained from the drainage bag of a Foley catheter closed drainage system.

   ❑ True

   ❑ False

7. Mr. Jacobson, a 78-year-old emphysemic, has been admitted for bacterial pneumonia. As part of the treatment plan he is receiving a medicated nebulizer treatment q 4 hours. The physician's order reads, "ABGs post nebulizer treatment." When would you have the ABGs drawn?

    a. Immediately after the treatment

    b. 15 minutes after the treatment

    c. 30 minutes after the treatment

8. What is the purpose of routine Heparin solution instillation in an unused port of a central line catheter?

    a. To prevent blood clots from forming in the catheter lumen

    b. To prevent the growth of microorganisms in the tubing

    c. To prevent analytes from forming in the tubing

    d. To prevent clotting in the specimen obtained from the port

9. The first void of a 24-hour urine specimen collection is discarded.

    ❏ True

    ❏ False

10. Ingestion of salicylates decreases prothrombin time (PT).

    ❏ True

    ❏ False

11. Which of the following diagnostic tests measures the intrinsic clotting mechanism factors (I, II, V, XI, XII)?

    a. PTT

    b. PT

    c. Thrombin time

12. Which of the following is a plasma protein that requires Vitamin K for synthesis?

    a. Prothrombin

    b. Thrombin

    c. Fibrinogen

    d. Platelets

13. The physician orders a "CBC with differential." When you are filling out the lab slip, which of the following should you check off?

    a. CBC and lymphocytes

    b. CBC and platelets

    c. CBC and monocytes

    d. CBC and WBC

14. A client with a low hemoglobin and hematocrit would be suspected of blood loss.

    ❑ True

    ❑ False

15. When a client is to receive blood, a type and crossmatch are performed. What is the purpose of the crossmatch procedure?

    a. To determine the presence or absence of A or B antigens in the client's blood

    b. To determine if the Rh factor is present in the client's blood

    c. To determine the compatibility of the recipient's blood with the donor blood

    d. To determine if the Rh agglutinins are present in the donor blood

16. Would you expect a platelet count to be included in a series of screening laboratory tests for a patient suspected of a coagulation disorder?

    ❑ Yes

    ❑ No

17. The lab values return for your client, showing an elevated LDH_1 and elevated CPK_2 (MB). This is indicative of

    a. myocardial damage.

    b. liver damage.

    c. brain damage.

    d. kidney damage.

18. Your 75-year-old client's electrolyte panel results are as follows: Na = 147; K = 3.7; Cl = 98. Are these values within normal limits?

    ❑ Yes

    ❑ No

19. Your patient's bloodwork comes back from the lab. Among the results you note that the ESR (sed rate) is moderately elevated. What would this most likely be indicative of?

    a. A concomitant elevation in blood glucose

    b. Increased stomach acidity

    c. The presence of an inflammatory process

    d. A folic acid deficiency

20. Match the study in the left column with the organ or body system it examines in the right column.

    _____ angiography   a. Peritoneal cavity

    _____ lymphangiography   b. Heart

    _____ cholangiography   c. Blood vessels

    _____ cystography   d. Lymphatic system

    _____ intravenous pyelogram   e. Urinary system

    _____ myelography   f. Bladder

    _____ electrocardiogram   g. Biliary system

    _____ arthroscopy   h. Spinal cord

    _____ laparoscopy   i. Joint structures

    _____ proctosigmoidoscopy   j. Rectum and colon

Chapter 29   *Medication Administration*

1. Nurses are responsible for dispensing and administering medications.

    ❑ True

    ❑ False

2. Which of the following mandates established the United States Pharmacopeia (USP) and the National Formulary (NF) as the official bodies that establish drug standards in the United States?

    a. The Harrison Narcotic Act

    b. The Food, Drug, and Cosmetic Act

    c. The Pure Food and Drug Act

    d. The Kefauver-Harris Act

3. Narcotic analgesics, such as morphine, are considered Schedule C-I controlled substances.

    ❑ True

    ❑ False

4. The physician's order reads *Aspirin one tablet qd in am.* In the patient's medication drawer you find two tablets; one is labeled Acetylsalicylic acid 325 mg, and the other is labeled Ferrous Sulfate 324 mg. When you ask a nurse on your unit what the generic name is for Aspirin, she replies it is Acetylsalicylic acid. Is this the correct answer?

    ❑ Yes

    ❑ No

5. Match each term in the left column with its definition from the right column.

    _____ peak plasma level   a. maintenance blood level of a drug

    _____ onset of action   b. when the body begins to respond to a drug

    _____ drug plateau   c. highest blood concentration level of a drug

    _____ drug half-life   d. the time it takes the body to eliminate half of the blood concentration of a drug

6. As you administer Nifedipine 20 mg sublingually, which of the following instructions would you give your patient?

    a. Make sure you chew the medication thoroughly before you swallow.

    b. Wait a few minutes before you drink or eat anything.

    c. This medication is absorbed in your stomach; make sure you swallow it whole.

    d. This medication must be dissolved completely and swallowed quickly.

7. The medication order reads *Heparin 5000 u SQ b.i.d.* Where in the body will this medication be given?

    a. The dermis

    b. The muscle

    c. The fatty tissue

    d. The vein

8. The bioavailability of a medication administered IM is greater than that of the same medication administered IV.

    ❏ True

    ❏ False

9. Mrs. Cameron has been admitted to your unit with a leg ulcer that will not heal. You suspect that this is related to her diabetes. Her admission lab work shows that her blood glucose is elevated; however, you notice that her liver enzymes are also elevated. You notice that the physician has continued her standing medications without any changes. Should you be concerned about her abnormal liver enzymes?

    ❏ Yes

    ❏ No

10. Mr. Bassinger is to be discharged in the morning on Coumadin 5 mg po q.d. He asks you if it is OK to eat spinach salads on his therapeutic diet. How would you answer him?

    ❏ Yes

    ❏ No

11. Mrs. Kaplan is ordered Dorzolamide hydrochloride 1 gtt OU t.i.d. Where and when will you administer this medication?

    a. In the right eye, twice per day

    b. In both eyes, twice per day

    c. In the left eye, three times per day

    d. In both eyes, three times per day

12. The physician's order reads *Tylenol 1 tsp q 4h PRN Temp above 101°F.* The medicine cup is marked in milliliters only. How many ml will you pour?

    a. 2 ml

    b. 5 ml

    c. 10 ml

    d. 15 ml

13. A medication order reads *NPH insulin 12 u SC.* This is an example of a

    a. single-dose order.

    b. stat order.

    c. standing order.

    d. PRN order.

14. The medication order reads *Inapsine 0.625 mg IV push q 4–6h PRN for nausea/vomiting.* Your patient needs a dose. It comes supplied as 2.5mg per ml. How much would you give?

    a. 0.25 ml

    b. 0.50 ml

    c. 1.0 ml

    d. 1.5 ml

15. List the five rights of medication administration.

    1. _____

    2. _____

    3. _____

    4. _____

    5. _____

16. You notice the LPN assigned to your team just left a patient's room to answer a call light. As you enter the patient's room you notice that the LPN has left the patient's medications at the bedside. The patient asks you, "Are these medications for me?" You answer "yes" and hand them to her. Is this safe practice?

    ❑ Yes

    ❑ No

17. Your assigned patient is receiving all medications via a PEG tube. The MAR reads *Enteric Coated ASA 1 tablet qd via tube.* What is the best course of action by the nurse?

    a. Crush the tablet, dissolve it, and administer via the PEG tube.

    b. Call the pharmacy to see if a liquid substitution is available.

    c. Contact the physician to clarify the order.

18. Which of the following needle gauges represents the largest needle diameter?

    a. 25 gauge

    b. 20 gauge

    c. 19 gauge

19. The medication administration Kardex reads *Neupogen 300 mcg SC qd.* Neupogen is supplied as 300mcg per ml. Which of the following syringes would you select to properly administer this medication?

    a. 1 ml tuberculin syringe with a 27 gauge needle

    b. 3 ml hypodermic syringe with a 20 gauge needle

    c. 3 ml hypodermic syringe with a 25 gauge needle

    d. 0.5 ml hypodermic syringe with a 27 gauge needle

20. An injectable medication that comes as a prefilled syringe is considered a unit dose.

    ❑ True

    ❑ False

21. Four milliliters is the largest volume that can be injected into a large muscle of an adult.

    ❑ True

    ❑ False

22. Is it acceptable to recap a used needle in order to transport it?

    ❑ Yes

    ❑ No

23. From which of the following containers would you use a filtered needle to withdraw medication?

    a. Ampule

    b. Multidose vial

    c. Single-dose vial

    d. Prefilled syringe

24. When administering an IV piggyback medication through a gravity flow system, the primary solution bag is lowered, via extension hook, prior to the start of the medication infusion. What is the rationale for this action?

    a. Ensures that no air will enter the secondary set tubing

    b. Reduces the risk of microorganisms entering the primary line tubing

    c. Allows the primary solution to continue infusing during the medication administration

    d. An increased hydrostatic pressure in the secondary bag causes the primary solution to stop flowing

25. Which of the following nursing considerations is critical when delivering medications IV push?

    a. The time interval to inject the drug

    b. The port of the IV tubing used to place the medication

    c. The time it takes for the drug to be absorbed

    d. The age of the patient

26. While you are assisting your client in using his metered-dose inhaler, he asks, "Why do I have to shake it before I use it?" Which of the following responses would correctly explain this to him?

    a. It makes sure that the two medications are mixed properly.

    b. It activates the medication.

    c. It allows for the medication to mix with the aerosol propellant.

Chapter 30 Responding to the Needs of the Perioperative Client

1. In which of the following types of surgical interventions would a surgeon *not* be able to discuss the setting and scheduling of the client's surgery?

    a. Emergency surgery

    b. Urgent surgery

    c. Elective surgery

2. Match the surgical intervention in the left column with its purpose from the right column.

    _____ diagnostic

    _____ reconstructive

    _____ curative

    _____ palliative

    _____ transplant

    a. Remove diseased tissue or organ and replace it with functioning tissue or organ

    b. Decrease the spread of a disease process to prolong life or to alleviate pain

    c. Repair or remove a diseased organ or restore normal physiological functioning

    d. Determine the origin of presenting symptoms and the extent of a disease process

    e. Correct a disease process or improve a cosmetic appearance

3. Most preoperative clients who will receive general anesthesia during surgery are required to have a chest X-ray.

    ❏ True

    ❏ False

4. Match the type of anesthesia in the left column with its effects from the right column.

_____ general anesthesia
    a. Temporary decreased sensation or loss of feeling and movement to the lower part of the body; drug injected through a needle or catheter placed directly into the spinal canal

_____ regional anesthesia
    b. Temporary loss of feeling or movement of an extremity; drug injected into veins of arm or leg

_____ major/minor nerve block
    c. Total unconscious state administered through inhalation or injection

_____ intravenous regional anesthesia
    d. Temporary loss of feeling or movement to a specific limb or area of the body; drug injected near multiple nerves or plexus

5. The nurse has the primary responsibility to screen a preoperative client for a previous episode of malignant hyperthermia during a prior surgery.

❑ True

❑ False

6. Halothane is a commonly used local anesthetic agent.

❑ True

❑ False

7. Which of the following is an appropriate nursing intervention after a client has been anesthetized with an oral anesthetic solution such as viscous lidocaine?

a. Rinse the mouth with saline solution until sensation returns.

b. Offer foods of puddinglike consistency until swallowing returns.

c. Keep the client NPO until the gag reflex returns.

d. Do not offer the client hot liquids until sensation returns.

8. Would you agree or disagree with the following statement? It is important to interview a presurgical client for the use of herbs because some herbal products interfere with anesthetic agents.

❑ Agree

❑ Disagree

9. Which of the following drugs places the client at risk for intra- and postoperative bleeding?

   a. Aspirin (non-narcotic analgesic, antipyretic)

   b. Prednisone (steroid)

   c. Sominex (bromide in comination)

   d. Amitriptyline (antidepressant)

10. Which of the following statements best explains the reason for performing and documenting the results of a nursing preoperative physical assessment?

    a. It is a requirement of the hospital.

    b. It provides a baseline for comparison of postoperative findings.

    c. It assists the nurse in beginning discharge planning.

    d. It replaces the physician's physical examination in some surgery centers.

11. Match the perioperative phase in the left column with the nursing diagnosis from the right column that is most likely to be relevant to clients within that perioperative phase.

    _____ preoperative

    _____ intraoperative

    _____ postoperative

    a. Anxiety related to risk factors related to surgery and anesthesia

    b. Ineffective airway clearance related to anesthesia

    c. Risk for injury related to positioning

12. Of the following preoperative procedures, which would you *not* expect to see on a preoperative checklist?

    a. Nail polish and make-up removal

    b. Lab work complete and on the chart

    c. Assessment of the patient's anxiety level

    d. Addressograph plate and MAR on the chart

13. The purpose of holding an inspiration for three seconds during the use of an incentive spirometer is to promote maximum chest contraction.

    ❑ True

    ❑ False

14. A blood clot or air that moves in the circulatory system from its place of origin is called a(n) _____.

15. The recommended frequency for removal of antiembolism stockings is

    a. once a day.

    b. twice a day.

    c. three times a day.

    d. twice in 8 hours.

16. For which of the following types of postoperative management equipment would a nurse be concerned about the lockout interval?

    a. TENS unit

    b. PCA pump

    c. ICD pump

    d. CPM machine

17. Match the surgical team member in the left column with the role of that member from the right column.

    _____ anesthetist   a. Obtains the surgical consent

    _____ surgeon   b. Obtains supplies and delivers materials in the operating room

    _____ first assistant   c. Prepares the instrument tray and passes the instruments to the surgeon

    _____ scrub nurse   d. Performs intubation prior to the beginning of surgery

    _____ circulating nurse   e. Helps the surgeon ligate, suction, and suture

18. OSHA standards require surgical personnel to comply with safety precautions while in the surgical arena. A 1999 study by Akdumann revealed that one-fourth of personnel wore no eye protection.

    ❑ True

    ❑ False

19. Patients are at high risk for injury related to hypothermia during surgery. Which of the following contributes to bodily heat loss?

    a. Anesthetic agents

    b. Exposure of large operative sites

    c. Exposure to a cold operating room

    d. All of the above

20. Which of the following incisions would you expect to find on a postoperative patient who had a splenectomy (spleen removal)?

    a. Left oblique subcostal

    b. Thoracoabdominal

    c. Lower vertical midline

    d. Upper vertical midline

21. The respiratory system receives priority during the initial postoperative nursing assessment.

    ❏ True

    ❏ False

22. Which of the following is an *abnormal* postoperative nursing assessment finding?

    a. Urinary output of less than 30cc per hour

    b. Pulse oximeter reading of 96%

    c. Absent bowel sounds

    d. Negative Homan's sign

23. Which of the following best describes the postoperative complication atelectasis?

    a. It is a lower level of oxygen in the blood.

    b. Pulmonary secretions pool which leads to decreased pulmonary ventilation.

    c. It is caused by a blood clot in the lungs which results in pulmonary obstruction.

    d. Inflammation of a vein causes pain and discomfort in the lower extremities.

24. Which of the following would you expect a postoperative client to be able to do at the time of discharge?

    a. Take own vital signs

    b. Relate symptoms to be reported to physician

    c. Create a two-week meal plan for a low-cholesterol diet

    d. Change a complex dressing using sterile technique

25. Mrs. Thompson, a two-day postthyroidectomy patient, is ambulatory around the unit, taking fluids, eating sparingly, and is unable to fully cooperate with deep breathing and coughing exercises because of incisional pain. Which of the following nursing diagnoses would receive priority for Mrs. Thompson?

    a. Altered nutrition: less than body requirements

    b. Ineffective airway clearance

    c. Risk for infection

    d. Acute pain

Chapter 31 Safety, Infection Control, and Hygiene

1. Match the terms in the left column with their definitions from the right column.

_____	pathogenicity	a.	Bacteria, viruses, fungi, protozoa, *Rickettsia*
_____	pathogens	b.	Something that is capable of causing disease
_____	virulence	c.	A plant or animal that harbors and provides sustenance for another organism
_____	infection	d.	Microorganisms acquired from environmental contact
_____	resident flora	e.	The degree to which a pathogen can produce disease
_____	transient flora	f.	Ability of a microorganism to produce disease
_____	host	g.	Invasion of a body tissue by microorganisms that results in cellular injury
_____	agent	h.	Always present, usually nonharmful microorganisms

2. Match each term in the left column with its definition from the right column.

_____	antigen	a.	Released by T-cells, attracts phagocytes and lymphocytes
_____	antibody	b.	Protein substances that counteract the effects of autogenic toxics
_____	lymphokines	c.	A substance that causes an antibody to form
_____	humoral immunity	d.	Stimulation of B-cells and antibody production
_____	acquired immunity	e.	The formation of memory B-cells, protects the host from the invasion of microbes

3. Place the following stages of infection in the proper sequence from invasion to recovery from the infection.

    _____ Illness

    _____ Prodromal

    _____ Convalescence

    _____ Incubation

4. Which of the following infections are health care workers most at risk to acquire?

    a. HIV

    b. HBV

    c. Lyme disease

    d. Abscess

5. Work-related back pain affects 38% of nurses.

    ❑ True

    ❑ False

6. What do the microorganisms VRE, MSRA, and MDRTB have in common?

    a. They are transmitted only in the droplet form.

    b. They are common drug-resistant nosocomial infections.

    c. They are uropathogens.

    d. They tend to invade immune intact hosts.

7. While delivering care you notice that you have developed a rash around your wrists and on the back of your hands. You suspect that you have developed an allergic contact dermatitis from the latex gloves used in your facility. Which of the following is your best course of action?

    a. Avoid coming in direct contact with the products containing latex until you are further evaluated by a physician.

    b. Continue to use the latex gloves and use a good handwashing technique.

8. Which of the following describes the first stage of the inflammatory process?

    a. Increased blood flow to the damaged area

    b. Infiltration of leukocytes into the damaged area

    c. Leakage of large amounts of plasma into the damaged area

    d. Release of chemicals

9. The recommended duration for handwashing during routine care is

    a. 5–10 seconds.

    b. 10–15 seconds.

    c. 15–20 seconds.

    d. 20–25 seconds.

10. The rate of nosocomial infections decreased in the years from 1975 to 1995.

    ❑ True

    ❑ False

11. Your client's ESR and WBC with differential lab results return. You note that the ESR and the neutrophil count are elevated. The eosinophil and monocyte counts are WNL. Do these lab results indicate that your client has an infection?

    ❑ Yes

    ❑ No

12. Which of the following nursing interventions is a priority for a patient at risk for falls?

    a. Provide adequate hydration and nutrition.

    b. Keep the bed in the lowest possible position.

    c. Place the patient in a room near the nurses' station.

    d. Offer the bedpan q 2h while the patient is in bed.

13. Your assigned patient, Mrs. Higgenbotham, is experiencing respiratory symptoms from an unknown source. Her physician has placed her on "droplet precautions." Which of the following precautions would you take when instituting droplet precautions?

    a. Gloves and gowns when in contact with the patient

    b. Gloves, gowns, and the use of a mask within 3 feet of the patient

    c. A private room and use of a HEPA filtered mask when in the patient's room

    d. A private room and the use of a mask within 3 feet of the patient

14. Place the following steps of bathing an adult in sequence from the beginning to the end of the bath.

    _____ Document skin assessment, type of bath, and client response.

    _____ Wash back.

    _____ Apply lotion or powder, then gown.

    _____ Place bath blanket over client.

    _____ Wash face.

    _____ Wash arms and hands.

    _____ Wash perineal area.

    _____ Wash legs and feet.

    _____ Wash chest and abdomen.

    _____ Obtain bath water.

15. A type A fire extinguisher will control any type of fire.

    ❑ True

    ❑ False

Chapter 32 Oxygenation

1. Mr. Priestly, who is one day post a lobectomy, has his oxygen saturation checked via a pulse oximeter every shift. Your finding is an O_2 saturation of 90% on 4L of oxygen via nasal cannula. How would this finding be interpreted?

   a. It is within normal limits.

   b. It is on the high end of normal for hemoglobin oxygenation.

   c. It is a low finding for a patient receiving oxygen.

2. Patients who experience tachycardia with heart rates above 130 with preexisting ventricular muscle weakness can experience a decrease in cardiac output due to which of the following factors?

   a. Loss of "atrial kick"

   b. An alteration in the cardiac conduction system

   c. A shift in the oxygen hemoglobin dissociation curve to the right

   d. Loss of atrial contractility

3. A client who experiences a collection of blood in the pleural space is experiencing which of the following conditions?

   a. Pneumothorax

   b. Pleural effusion

   c. Chlyothorax

   d. Hemothorax

4. Mr. Briggs is in your care because he has experienced an exacerbation of his congestive heart failure (CHF) and his physician suspects he may have pneumonia. When you auscultate his lungs, which breath sound would you expect to hear that would most accurately reflect his unresolved CHF? _____.

5. Which of the following medications would be indicated to promote bronchial dilation and increase ciliary movement?

   a. Cromolyn Sodium

   b. Aminophylline

   c. Beclomethasone

   d. Mucomyst

6. Mr. Jameson has a history of chronic obstructive pulmonary disease with acute substernal chest pain. He has been admitted to the intensive care unit for observation as well as to rule out a myocardial infarction. Which of the following tests performed on Mr. Jameson would inform the nurse of the extent to which he is experiencing air trapping?

   a. Sputum sample analysis

   b. Arterial blood gas analysis

   c. Electrocardiography

   d. Ventilation scan

7. Clubbing of the nailbed is a result of chronic hypoxia.

   ❑ True

   ❑ False

8. Prolonged administration of a high $Fi\,O_2$ can damage lung tissue.

   ❑ True

   ❑ False

9. Mrs. Thatcher presents in the emergency room with a chief complaint of pain in her right lower chest and states she is having difficulty "catching her breath." Which of the following open-ended questions would be most useful during the focal interview to elicit additional information about her presenting problem?

   a. How many packs of cigarettes a day do you smoke?

   b. Describe the pain for me.

   c. Tell me what you have had to eat today.

   d. Can you describe your medical history?

10. Mr. Smith has a nursing order on his care plan to suction his tracheostomy tube PRN. Which of the following assessments will indicate that he needs suctioning?

   a. His breath sounds are diminished.

   b. He is unable to perform deep breathing and coughing exercises.

   c. There is collection of moisture in the oxygen tubing, creating a bubbling sound.

   d. You hear gurgling noises when he breathes.

11. A common nursing diagnosis for a postoperative patient is *Risk for Ineffective Airway Clearance*. Which of the following interventions would *not* be appropriate for a patient with this potential problem?

   a. Restricting fluid intake

   b. Splinting incision during respiratory hygiene measures

   c. Chest physiotherapy every 2–4 hours

   d. Incentive spirometer every 1–2 hours

   e. Deep breathing and coughing every 1–2 hours

12. A common cause of impaired gas exchange when there is evidence of alveolar collapse is called _____.

13. What is the maximum time suction should be applied to the respiratory mucosa?

   a. 3–5 seconds

   b. 6–9 seconds

   c. 10–15 seconds

   d. 16–20 seconds

14. Ms. Jones, a 16-year-old, has just been admitted to the Pediatric Unit with chronic diarrhea and vomiting and shortness of breath. She has an IV of D_5W infusing at 125 cc per hour and oxygen at 2L per minute via nasal cannula. The nurse technician comes to you and asks if the oxygen should be humidified. How would you answer?

   ❑ Yes

   ❑ No

15. Which of the following is the appropriate amount of suction to use when performing oropharyngeal suctioning?

   a. 80 mm Hg

   b. 90 mm Hg

   c. 100 mm Hg

   d. 110 mm Hg

Chapter 33   Comfort and Sleep

1. Pain is an objective, measurable experience.
   - ❏ True
   - ❏ False

2. Which of the following describes pain originating in the internal organs?
   - a. Visceral pain
   - b. Somatic pain
   - c. Cutaneous pain
   - d. Neuralgia

3. The changing of noxious stimuli in sensory nerve endings to energy impulses is referred to as
   - a. modulation.
   - b. transduction.
   - c. transmission.
   - d. perception.

4. The four vital signs are blood pressure, temperature, pulse, and respiration. Which of the following is now considered the "fifth" vital sign?
   - a. Comfort
   - b. Sleep
   - c. Hydration status
   - d. Pain level

5. For which of the following types of pain would oxygen administration be indicated?
   - a. Colic
   - b. Ischemic
   - c. Neuropathic
   - d. Myofascial

6. An expected finding for a client experiencing progressive pain is an elevation in pulse, respiratory rates, and blood pressure.

   ❑ True

   ❑ False

7. Which of the following nursing interventions have a basis in the gate control theory of pain management?

   a. Administering acetaminophen (Tylenol) as ordered

   b. Distracting the client with television

   c. Administering a back massage

   d. Allowing the client to express negative feelings

8. The threshold for experiencing pain varies according to type of pain and the individual response to that pain.

   ❑ True

   ❑ False

9. Mrs. Apperson, age 80, has had arthritis "as long as I can remember." She has difficulty ambulating and says it's because of her stiff, painful joints. She rates her pain most times as a 4 on a 10-point scale. She has gained 10 lbs. over the past two months. The staff has noticed that she doesn't ambulate as often as she used to; she says she is afraid of falling. Which of the following NANDA nursing diagnoses would be appropriate for Mrs. Apperson?

   a. Pain

   b. Chronic pain

   c. Acute pain

   d. Fatigue

10. What is the major advantage to the use of a PCA pump in pain management?

   a. The pharmacy prepares the medication.

   b. It is possible to administer more than the usual and customary dose of an analgesic.

   c. The Pain Management Team is responsible for accuracy of the dose prescription.

   d. The patient can control the dosing of the analgesic.

11. Match the pain intervention in the left column with its definition from the right column.

_____ distraction

_____ imagery

_____ biofeedback

_____ cryotherapy

_____ progressive muscle relaxation

_____ hypnosis

_____ TENS

_____ acupuncture

_____ acupressure

a. Application of heat and needles to various points on the body

b. Focuses the attention away from the pain

c. Clients learn to influence their physiologic responses

d. Release of blocked energy along certain pressure points on the body

e. Application of minute amounts of electrical stimulation to large-diameter nerve fibers

f. Cold application

g. Leads to a reduction in skeletal muscle tension

h. A state of heightened awareness and focused concentration

i. Focuses attention on a mental picture

12. PRN analgesic medication administration maintains a therapeutic serum level.

❑ True

❑ False

13. Which of the following is an advantage of using the intravenous versus subcutaneous opioid infusion as a route of medication administration?

a. There is no associated tissue volume restriction.

b. There is less risk for infection to the insertion site.

c. It provides more effective pain relief.

d. It requires pharmacy support in order to deliver the medication.

14. Based on what you know about the "ceiling effect," which of the following statements would you make when educating family members about medicating a child with an analgesic?

a. If your child's pain is not affected by this medication, it is OK to increase the dose by half.

b. If your child's pain is not decreased by this medication, stop the medication and call the physician.

c. If your child's pain is not affected by this medication, do not increase the dose; the effect is the same, but the risk for experiencing side effects increases.

d. If your child's pain is not decreased by this medication, call the physician for a new medication prescription.

15. Match the term in the left column with its definition from the right column.

_____ addiction   a. Results in withdrawal symptoms when drug is stopped suddenly

_____ tolerance   b. Psychological dependence

_____ physical dependence   c. Client requires a larger dose of medication to achieve the same effect.

16. Jose Ortega, 12 years old, has been admitted to your pediatric unit after sustaining injuries in a motor vehicle accident (MVA). The physician order reads "Administer Morphine 6mg q 3h PRN for pain." Jose weighs 98 lbs. The recommended dosing for a child less than 50 kg is 0.1mg/kg q 3–4h. Is the ordered dose a safe dose?

❏ Yes

❏ No

17. EMLA® cream is an example of a topical anesthetic used to anesthetize the skin prior to intravenous catheter insertion.

❏ True

❏ False

18. Match the term in the left column with its definition from the right column.

_____ narcolepsy   a. Manifests by clients sleeping excessively

_____ hypersomnia   b. Pauses in breathing of 30–60 seconds during sleep

_____ sleep apnea   c. Grinding of the teeth during sleep

_____ sleep deprivation   d. Sleep walking

_____ somnambulism   e. Sudden uncontrollable urges to fall asleep during the day

_____ bruxism   f. Prolonged inadequacy of quality and quantity of sleep

19. Mrs. Chang, 78 years old, is admitted to your unit for an endocrine system evaluation. During the assessment interview you learn that she sleeps 6 hours a night. Should this be of concern?

❏ Yes

❏ No

20. The interventions on a care plan with the nursing diagnosis *Sleep Pattern Disturbance R/T pain* would focus on pain management.

❏ True

❏ False

Chapter **34** *Mobility*

1. Nurses are encouraged by their employers to use good body mechanics. What is meant by "good body mechanics"?

   a. Body parts in the proper position in relation to each other, allowing the body to maintain equilibrium

   b. The use of body parts and positions during activity in order to reduce strain

   c. The use of body parts and positions in order to maintain balance

2. Which of the following reflects the effects of immobility on the musculoskeletal system?

   a. Risk of thrombi formation

   b. Protein annabolism

   c. Calcium loss

   d. Increased respiratory capacity

3. Increased dietary protein is provided for patients who are immobile. Which of the following statements best explains the reason for this intervention?

   a. This is an attempt at the prevention of pressure ulcers.

   b. Negative nitrogen balance occurs.

   c. Peristalsis decreases; therefore, patients lose their appetites.

   d. There is a tendency for the immobile to form renal calculi.

4. Mrs. Cassidy was admitted earlier this morning with a cerebrovascular accident, with her right side affected. She is confused and she cannot feed herself or wash herself. Based on these assessment data, which of the following nursing diagnoses is the most appropriate for Mrs. Cassidy?

   a. Self-care deficits

   b. Impaired physical mobility

   c. Activity intolerance

   d. Risk for aspiration

5. While ambulating Mr. Jones, you encourage him to stand and walk using good body posture. Which of the following instructions would you give him?

   a. Stand with your back straight.

   b. Tuck your abdominal muscles in.

   c. Walk with your head up, face forward.

   d. All of these instructions.

6. Match each term from the left column with its definition from the right column.

   _____ active ROM   a. Bending of the joint so that articulating bones are moved farther apart

   _____ passive ROM   b. One body part being across another body part at least 180 degrees

   _____ active-assistive ROM   c. ROM performed by the client

   _____ adduction   d. ROM performed by the nurse

   _____ supination   e. Turning the body or body part upward

   _____ opposition   f. Moving toward the midline

   _____ extension   g. ROM performed by the client, nurse assists

7. The purpose for placing a lift sheet under a patient who needs to be lifted up in bed is to reduce the shearing force that occurs when a patient is moved up in bed.

   ❑ True

   ❑ False

8. You hear in report that the head of Mr. Winkler's bed is to be kept in high Fowler's position. In which of the following angle elevations would you expect to find the patient?

   a. 30 degrees

   b. 45 degrees

   c. 60 degrees

   d. 75 degrees

9. Which of the following types of exercise would you advise a patient with a cardiovascular problem to avoid?

    a. Isometric

    b. Aerobic

    c. Isotonic

    d. Isokinetic

10. Which of the following misalignments of the spine would you expect to find during an assessment of an elderly female client?

    a. Scoliosis

    b. Lordosis

    c. Kyphosis

    d. List

11. Which of the following assessments is *not* common to both skeletal and skin traction?

    a. Body position

    b. Traction weights

    c. Traction rope

    d. Appearance of pin or wire site

12. The patient care technician comes to you and asks, "How do I walk Mr. Haggedorn? He has a chest tube drain going." How will you respond?

    a. Disconnect the chest drainage system from the patient; put a 4×4 gauze dressing over the chest tube and pin it to his gown. Reconnect it when he returns to his room.

    b. Disconnect the drainage system from the wall suction, put the system on a cart, keeping it upright, ambulate him, then rehook it to the suction when he returns to his room.

    c. You can't ambulate him; he has a chest tube in.

13. Wheelchair brakes should be locked prior to transferring a client in or out of a wheelchair.

    ❑ True

    ❑ False

14. Mr. Dickens is comatose. You ask Mrs. Dickens to bring in a pair of high-topped sneakers for Mr. Dickens. She asks, "What good will they do?" How will you respond?

    a. He will need them when he regains consciousness.

    b. They will relieve pressure on his heels.

    c. They will help prevent foot drop.

    d. They will improve circulation to his feet.

15. The maximum number of hours a client should stay in one position is _____.

16. When lifting an object, bend at the knees, not the waist. What is the principle behind this practice of good body mechanics?

    a. It provides a stable base to lift from.

    b. It is a more comfortable posture.

    c. It provides greater leverage for lifting.

    d. It supports the back muscles.

17. An example of a ball and socket joint is the elbow.

    ❏ True

    ❏ False

18. Which of the following crutch gaits is used when one leg is non–weight bearing?

    a. Four-point

    b. Three-point

    c. Two-point

    d. Swing-through

19. The following are all factors that, when combined, could place a client at risk for falls. According to the Risk Assessment Tool for Falls, which of these factors *alone* places the client at risk for a fall?

    a. Urinary frequency

    b. Vision impairment

    c. Confusion

    d. Use of a cane

20. Mrs. Duncan was admitted yesterday with degenerative joint disease as a result of her long history of arthritis. Today she had a right total hip replacement (THR). The postanesthesia care unit nurse tells you in report that Mrs. Duncan's hip needs to remain in neutral position. An abductor pillow is in place. What is the purpose of the abductor pillow?

   a. To improve the circulation to the surgical area

   b. To immobilize the hip joint

   c. To ensure that the affected leg does not move laterally

   d. To prevent the right hip from the flexion and extension movement

Chapter 35   *Skin Integrity and Wound Healing*

1. Wound healing occurs in three phases. In which of the following phases does collagen deposition occur?

   a. Defensive

   b. Reconstructive

   c. Maturation

2. Match the term in the left column with its definition from the right column.

   _____ phagocytosis   a. Includes new blood vessels and connective tissue

   _____ exudate   b. Formation of blood vessels

   _____ granulation tissue   c. Necrotic tissue

   _____ angiogenesis   d. Envelopment and destruction of microorganisms by leukocytes

   _____ hematoma   e. Collection of blood under the skin

   _____ eschar   f. Fluid and other material that accumulates in wounds

3. Mr. Sullivan is three days out of surgery. During the dressing change you notice that the drainage is thick and yellow and the wound edges, previously approximated, are beginning to separate. Which of the following terms best labels this drainage?

   a. Serous

   b. Purulent

   c. Sanguineous

   d. Serosanguineous

4. The role of Vitamin C in wound healing is to support capillary formation and stabilization.

   ❑ True

   ❑ False

5. Mrs. Hayes, 37 years old, is admitted for a debridement of a leg ulcer that has not healed in two months. During her admission interview you learn that she is a diabetic, she follows her diabetic diet, and is able to perform all ADLs. She is a nonsmoker and takes her diabetic (glyburide) and her blood pressure (amlodipine) medications without interruption. Which of the following factors most likely plays a role in the delay of Mrs. Hayes's wound healing?

    a. Age

    b. Blood pressure medication

    c. Diabetes

    d. Nutritional status

6. Skin loss that is confined to epidermal tissue is called a

    a. first-degree wound.

    b. second-degree wound.

    c. third-degree wound.

7. Mr. Church had abdominal surgery four days ago. He puts his call light on and states to the unit secretary, "Something's popped in my belly." Upon inspection you find his wound has eviscerated. Which of the following interventions would you immediately carry out?

    a. Call his surgeon and the OR.

    b. Apply a dry sterile dressing.

    c. Apply a sterile, saline-soaked dressing.

    d. Apply pressure using a sterile dressing.

8. During report you learn that Mrs. Richards has been admitted with a second-degree burn to her left forearm. How would you expect the wound to appear when you do her assessment?

    a. Red and dry

    b. Red and blistery with swelling and exudate

    c. Red and crusty with some blackened areas

9. Which of the following types of drainage systems is a Hemovac drain an example of?

    a. Closed suction

    b. Open gravity

10. Which of the following lab values would you consult to learn what protein reserves are available for wound healing?

    a. Albumin

    b. WBC

    c. RBC

    d. Cholesterol

11. For which of the following clients would a nurse be on the alert for a risk for injury when applying a hot pack?

    a. A 5-year-old with an infection under the fingernail

    b. A 45-year-old cardiac-diseased client with an IV infiltrate

    c. An 80-year-old diabetic with a wound infection

12. Todd Masters, a 4-year-old, comes into the emergency room with a laceration to his head. He is bleeding profusely (as head wounds do) and crying out in pain. You cleanse the wound and place a sterile gauze dressing over it. While he is waiting for the physician, which type of therapy would you place over the dressing?

    a. An Aqua K pad (aquathermia unit)

    b. A warm washcloth

    c. An ice bag

    d. A cold, wet compress

13. When cleansing a surgical wound, in which direction would you stroke the incision?

    a. Toward the incision

    b. Away from the incision

14. Which of the following irrigation solutions would be most appropriate for cleansing an infected wound?

    a. Full-strength hydrogen peroxide

    b. Full-strength Provo-iodine

    c. Sterile saline

    d. Half-strength hydrogen peroxide

15. Mr. McGowan is status post coronary artery bypass graft surgery. He has been readmitted to your unit after undergoing a debridement of his infected sternal wound. The surgeon has left the wound open and has ordered wet to dry saline dressing changes q.i.d. Which of the following types of wound healing is this considered?

    a. Primary intention healing

    b. Secondary intention healing

    c. Tertiary intention healing

16. Which of the following interventions would be appropriate on a nursing care plan when a client is at high risk for skin breakdown?

    a. Massage bony prominances four times a day.

    b. Use alcohol during back rubs; perform three times a day.

    c. Turn and reposition every 2 hours.

    d. Place a donut on the wheelchair seat while client is up in the wheelchair.

17. Which of the following moisture-retentive dressings would you use for a Stage II pressure ulcer which has moderate amounts of drainage?

    a. Transparent adhesive (e.g., Tegaderm)

    b. Hydrogel (e.g., Carrasyn Hydrogel Wound Dressing)

    c. Exudate absorber (e.g., Debrisan)

    d. Hydrocolloid (e.g., DuoDERM)

18. You remove an IV cannula from a patient's infiltrated IV site and direct a nurse's aide to apply a warm compress to this site. You should direct the aide to leave the compress on for what length of time?

    a. 10 minutes

    b. 20 minutes

    c. 40 minutes

    d. 60 minutes

19. When packing a wound with moist dressing material, the wound should be packed tightly.

    ❏ True

    ❏ False

20. Which of the following assessments is a predictor of skin breakdown?

    a. Stage II pressure ulcer

    b. Persistent erythma of the skin

    c. Blanching when pressure is applied to the skin

    d. Ischemia

Chapter **36** *Sensation, Perception, and Cognition*

1. Which of the following parts of the brain is responsible for maintaining equilibrium?

    a. Cerebrum

    b. Brain stem

    c. Cerebellum

    d. Broca's area

2. Afferent nerve pathways carry sensory impulses away from the brain.

    ❑ True

    ❑ False

3. Which of the following controls sleep/wakefulness and consciousness?

    a. The glossopharyngeal nerve

    b. The somatic nervous system

    c. The diencephalon

    d. The reticular activating system

4. A client states, "The president of the United States is telling me that I must leave this place." This statement is an example of

    a. an illusion.

    b. a visual hallucination.

    c. an auditory hallucination.

    d. poor judgment.

5. Which of the following situations would place a client at risk for developing sensory overload?

    a. A 10-year-old in the X-ray department waiting for a chest X-ray

    b. A 79-year-old in the intensive care unit recovering from surgery

    c. A 40-year-old, with a chief complaint of a skin rash, being evaluated by a nurse practitioner

    d. An 85-year-old receiving a vitamin injection in her home by a visiting nurse

6. Mrs. Provencano, a 90-year-old resident in your long-term care facility, is hard of hearing, cannot ambulate, and speaks Italian with very few words of English. Her daughter visits rarely because of distance. Her daughter states that her mother feels alone now that most of her friends have died and her family can't visit as much as she desires. Which of the following nursing diagnoses would best apply for Mrs. Provencano?

    a. Social Isolation

    b. Altered Thought Process

    c. Sensory-Perceptual Alteration: Hearing

    d. Ineffective Family Coping

7. You assess Mr. Jones's mental status. He can tell you his name but not what day it is or where he is. He knows he has been ill but cannot tell you the reason for his admission. Which of the following nurses' notes would be an accurate documentation of his orientation?

    a. Oriented × 1

    b. Oriented × 2

    c. Oriented × 3

8. Prolonged understimulation can result in disorientation.

    ❑ True

    ❑ False

9. As you listen to report on your patient, Mr. Lee, you hear that his level of consciousness (LOC) has deteriorated from alert to obtunded. Based on this information, how would you expect to find him when you enter his room?

    a. Nonverbal, unable to follow commands, but does move if stimulated

    b. Unconscious with no meaningful response to stimuli

    c. Slow to respond, drifts off to sleep when not stimulated

    d. Sleeps most of the time, inconsistently follows commands, difficult to arouse

10. Which of the following would you teach a client who is experiencing a tactile deficit?

    a. Use assistive devices such as a hearing aid.

    b. Place a calendar and clock in rooms that you frequent.

    c. Avoid using heating pads.

    d. Purchase books on tape or books that contain large print.

11. As the charge RN in your long-term care facility, a nurse's aide comes to you and asks if a confused resident can take a shower independently. How would you respond to this aide?

    ❑ Yes

    ❑ No

12. All procedures should be explained to an unconscious client.

    ❑ True

    ❑ False

13. You have placed the nursing diagnosis *Disturbed Thought Process* on Mr. Jubinski's care plan. Which of the following nursing interventions is appropriate to include on his care plan?

    a. Keep the environment calm.

    b. Monitor client closely; check every 30 minutes.

    c. Use physical restraints PRN.

    d. Participate in large-group activities as often as possible.

14. Which of the following nursing diagnoses is a priority for a client who is experiencing an altered level of consciousness?

    a. Sensory-Perceptual Alteration

    b. Risk for Injury

    c. Disturbed Thought Process

    d. Disturbed Body Image

15. Which of the following interventions would be appropriate for a client experiencing a visual impairment?

    a. Use brief, concise statements.

    b. Speak in raised tones.

    c. Keep objects in their usual place.

    d. Provide a private room whenever possible.

16. A score of 6 on the Glascow Coma Scale (GCS) would indicate that a client is fully alert and oriented.

    ❑ True

    ❑ False

17. You are assessing Mrs. Tatro. She cannot remember if her daughter was in to visit her yesterday. She *can* remember, with clarity, events from her early adulthood. How would you summarize the quality of her memory?

    a. Recent recall but poor long-term memory

    b. Intact long-term memory but limited recent recall

    c. Intact long-term memory but poor immediate memory

18. A commonly used nursing intervention is patient teaching. Which of the following statements best supports the strategy to delay patient teaching when a patient's anxiety level is high?

    a. As the anxiety level increases, it interferes with the patient's ability to concentrate by decreasing his or her attention span.

    b. During high anxiety periods, efferent nerve pathways are stimulated which causes a disruption in memory.

19. You read on the client's medical record that the client has "poor impulse control." For which of the following components of cognition does this entry reflect an assessment?

    a. Affect

    b. Judgment

    c. Perception

    d. Memory

20. Which of the following medications would *not* contribute to the alteration in level of consciousness?

    a. Morphine Sulfate (analgesic)

    b. Librium (Benzodiazepine)

    c. Phenobarbital (sedative)

    d. Insulin (antidiabetic agent)

Chapter 37 Fluid, Electrolyte, and Acid-Base Balance

1. Match the term in the left column with its definition from the right column.

    _____ solute

    _____ solvent

    _____ electrolyte

    _____ body fluid

    a. The liquid that contains a substance in solution

    b. The substance that dissociates into ions when dissolved

    c. A solution that contains both electrolytes and water

    d. The substance dissolved in a solution

2. Which of the following is the most frequently occurring intracellular cation?

    a. Na^+

    b. K^+

    c. Ca^{++}

    d. Mg^{++}

3. A function of the electrolyte sodium in the body is to

    a. provide strength and durability to the bones and teeth.

    b. regulate vascular osmotic pressure.

    c. regulate the osmolarity of intracellular fluid.

    d. activate enzyme systems within the body.

4. The force that presses outward against a blood vessel wall is

    a. colloid osmotic pressure.

    b. hydrostatic pressure.

    c. osmotic pressure.

    d. the rate of blood flow.

5. The lungs play a role in the regulation of fluid balance.

    ❑ True

    ❑ False

6. A solution with a pH of 7.46 is considered acidic.

   ❑ True

   ❑ False

7. Hypernatremia means that there is an excess of potassium ions in the ECF.

   ❑ True

   ❑ False

8. Mr. Canavan is admitted with a diagnosis of congestive heart failure (CHF) and has a history of insulin-dependent diabetes mellitus (IDDM). His medications include insulin, which he self-administers twice a day, as well as Lasix (furosemide), which he takes once a day orally. Your physical assessment findings reveal hypoactive bowel sounds, muscle weakness, and tachycardia. His admitting EKG shows an inverted T-wave. His wife reports his appetite has been diminished over the past few days. You conclude Mr. Canavan is

   a. hypokalemic.

   b. hyperkalemic.

   c. hypocalcemic.

   d. hypermagnesemic.

9. Ms. Miller is one day post surgery for removal of her thyroid. The nursing care plan indicates Ms. Miller's Chvostek's sign will be assessed each shift. A positive Chvostek's sign indicates

   a. hypocalcemia.

   b. hypercalcemia.

   c. hypokalemia.

   d. hyperphosphatemia.

10. Which of the following sources of laboratory data would you look at first if you suspected your client of having an acid-base imbalance?

    a. Arterial blood gases

    b. Hemoglobin and hematocrit

    c. Serum potassium

    d. Serum sodium

11. You review the lab reports for your client and find that the pH is high, the PaO$_2$ is normal, PCO$_2$ is normal, and the HCO$_3$ is high. This indicates

    a. metabolic alkalosis.

    b. metabolic acidosis.

    c. respiratory acidosis.

    d. respiratory alkalosis.

12. Edema documented as +2 means the client's edema is moderate.

    ❑ True

    ❑ False

13. The osmolarity of the IV solution D$_5$ in .45 saline is

    a. hypotonic.

    b. isotonic.

    c. hypertonic.

14. The proper method to assess skin turgor is to pinch and release the skin over the sternum of an adult.

    ❑ True

    ❑ False

15. The proper infusion rate of IV potassium chloride is 30 mEq per hour.

    ❑ True

    ❑ False

16. Which of the following assessments most accurately determines a client's fluid status?

    a. Daily weights

    b. 24-hour intake and output calculations

    c. Assessment of vital signs q 8 hours

17. Patients who are NPO should receive mouth care every 1–2 hours. Would the use of glycerin mouth swabs be a good choice when providing mouth care?

    ❑ Yes

    ❑ No

18. Mrs. Sandler is two days postoperative a left mastectomy (removal of breast). Her IV has been infiltrated and you need to restart her IV. Which extremity would you select to restart the IV?

    a. Left arm

    b. Right arm

19. The physician's order reads: "250cc's Normal Saline IV, infuse over 3 hours." The drop factor of the macrotubing is 15 gtts/ml. How many drops per minute will this gravity flow IV infuse?

    a. 15

    b. 21

    c. 40

    d. 83

20. Your patient has a primary IV infusing of D_5W at 125cc's per hour. The physician orders Ampicillin 250mg in 50cc of normal saline IVPB q.i.d. The primary and secondary IV are on a volume control pump. The pharmacy recommends the infusion be delivered in 30 minutes. At what flow rate will you program the secondary (the IVPB) pump?

    a. 50cc per hour

    b. 100cc per hour

    c. 150cc per hour

    d. 200cc per hour

21. Your patient is saying that his IV site is tender. Upon inspection you find that it is slightly pink and swollen 1–2 inches above the insertion site and it feels warm. These findings indicate

    a. phlebitis.

    b. infiltration.

    c. edema.

    d. thrombus.

22. Blood should be infused within 4 hours after initiating the transfusion. Which of the following statements best explains the rationale for the 4-hour limit?

    a. This elevates the hemoglobin and hematocrit levels.

    b. It provides for the client's comfort.

    c. It reduces the risk for the development of hyperkalemia.

    d. It minimizes the risk for the development of a transfusion reaction.

23. Which of the following solutions is appropriate to hang as a secondary bag of fluid to flush tubing that will deliver blood?

    a. Normal saline, 0.9%

    b. Ringer's lactate

    c. 0.45% saline

    d. D_5% in 0.45% saline

24. When prepping skin for venipuncture, the skin should be scrubbed with betadine followed by alcohol.

    ❑ True

    ❑ False

25. When air enters the primary tubing of an infusing IV, it is best removed by detaching the tubing from the needle and opening the clamp to allow fluid to clear the air out of the tubing.

    ❑ True

    ❑ False

26. Which of the following solutions does the Intravenous Nurses Society recommend to flush an intravenous cannula?

    a. Heparin

    b. Saline

27. Which of the following IV sites would be your first choice when starting an IV on a patient who has just been admitted?

    a. Dorsal plexus vein

    b. Median cubital vein

    c. Great saphenous vein

    d. Dorsal metacarpal vein

28. Why should you wear clean gloves when discontinuing an IV?

    a. The client and family expect this. It promotes psychological well-being.

    b. You minimize potential exposure to body fluids.

    c. You reduce the possibility of introducing microorganisms into the open IV insertion site.

29. Which of the following nursing diagnoses would be appropriate for a patient who has an IV infusing at KVO rate?

    a. Fluid Volume Deficit

    b. Risk for Infection

    c. Altered Oral Mucous Membranes

    d. Impaired Skin Integrity

30. Should you consider the size of the syringe you use when flushing a cannula?

    ❑ Yes

    ❑ No

Chapter 38 Nutrition

1. Which of the following is an inorganic nutrient?

   a. Water

   b. Vitamin

   c. Carbohydrate

   d. Protein

2. In a healthy adult, what percentage of total body weight is water?

   a. 20–30%

   b. 40–50%

   c. 50–60%

   d. 60–70%

3. Which of the following nutrients does pancreatic lipase act on in the digestive process?

   a. Carbohydrates

   b. Proteins

   c. Vitamins

   d. Fats

4. Which of the following minerals plays a role in the formation of thyroid hormone?

   a. Iodine

   b. Iron

   c. Copper

   d. Zinc

5. Megadoses of vitamins are recommended in the maintenance of health.

   ❑ True

   ❑ False

6. Match the vitamin in the left column with its function from the right column.

_____ Vitamin A   a. Prevents oxidation of polyunsaturated fatty acids

_____ Vitamin D   b. Promotes the metabolism of carbohydrates

_____ Vitamin E   c. Promotes the oxidation of carbohydrates, fats, and protein

_____ Vitamin K   d. Is a coenzyme to protein and carbohydrate metabolism

_____ Vitamin C   e. Supports retinal pigmentation

_____ Vitamin B1   f. Supports the production of collagen

_____ Vitamin B2   g. Plays a role in blood clotting

_____ Vitamin B6   h. Promotes bone and tooth development

7. During the interview, your client states that she read in the newspaper that anitoxidants are good for you. She asks, "Which vitamins can I take that have these antioxidants in them?" Which of the following is the correct response?

a. Vitamins A, C, and E

b. Vitamin B complex

c. Vitamins D and K

8. Excess glucose in the body is stored as glycogen in the

a. liver and muscles.

b. liver and pancreas.

c. muscles and brain.

d. fatty tissue and muscles.

9. If the body does not have enough carbohydrates, it begins to break down body proteins in order to produce energy. What is the minimum level of carbohydrate ingestion necessary to prevent protein breakdown?

a. 25–50 grams

b. 50–100 grams

c. 100–150 grams

d. 150–200 grams

10. What is the minimum amount of protein a person must ingest to prevent obligatory protein loss?

a. 5–10 grams

b. 10–20 grams

c. 20–30 grams

d. 30–40 grams

11. Low-density lipoproteins are responsible for the formation of atherosclerosis.
    ❑ True
    ❑ False

12. In some cultures, excess body weight is highly desirable.
    ❑ True
    ❑ False

13. Using the food groups listed, build the food pyramid from the base up.
    _____ Fats, oils, and sweets
    _____ Fruits and vegetables
    _____ Bread, cereal, rice, and pasta
    _____ Dairy products and meats

14. Ascites is indicative of protein deficiency.
    ❑ True
    ❑ False

15. Abdominal girth is assessed in order to evaluate the contour of the abdomen.
    ❑ True
    ❑ False

16. Your patient's lab results reveal an elevated BUN and normal serum creatinine. This indicates malnutrition.
    ❑ True
    ❑ False

17. It is estimated that 10% of hospitalized patients are at risk for malnutrition.
    ❑ True
    ❑ False

18. Which of the following assessments would indicate to a nurse that the client's diet could be progressed from a clear liquid to a full liquid diet? The client
    a. has hypoactive bowel sounds.
    b. has normal bowel sounds.
    c. reports nausea.
    d. is experiencing severe diarrhea.

19. Which of the following reflects a diet moderately restricted in sodium?

    a. 2000mg

    b. 1000mg

    c. 500mg

    d. 250mg

20. Which of the following clients would be a candidate for parenteral nutrition? A client who

    a. can only swallow thickened liquids.

    b. chokes when attempting to swallow foods or liquids.

    c. is experiencing an intestinal obstruction.

    d. consistently ingests 25% of food that is served.

21. Which of the following actions is the proper method to confirm placement of a small-bore feeding tube?

    a. Aspirate gastric contents with a Luer-Lok syringe and check the pH of the contents.

    b. Begin tube feeding which has been tinted with blue food coloring.

    c. Assess breath sounds.

    d. Assess abdominal sounds.

22. The radiologist calls you and states that the chest X-ray reveals that the small-bore feeding tube needs to be advanced 4 inches prior to initiating the tube feeding. You assess your patient and learn that the guidewire has been removed. Should you reinsert the guidewire before you take further action?

    ❑ Yes

    ❑ No

23. Your patient is ordered to receive intermittent bolus tube feedings q 4h. You aspirate the feeding tube and find that the gastric residual is 200cc. Which of the following actions would you take?

    a. Hold the tube feeding until the residual diminishes.

    b. Place the patient in low Fowler's position.

    c. Administer the bolus tube feeding.

    d. Administer the tube feeding continuously via pump.

24. The purpose of flushing a feeding tube q 4h with 30cc of water is to hydrate the patient.

    ❑ True

    ❑ False

25. Which of the following actions would be taken before hanging a subsequent bag of TPN?

    a. Draw the serum BUN and creatinine blood sample immediately prior to hanging the bag.

    b. Document the clotting times on the patient record prior to hanging the bag.

    c. Mix the lipids with the TPN prior to hanging the bag.

    d. Use new tubing and attach an IV filter prior to hanging the bag.

Chapter 39   Elimination

1. Match the term in the left column with its definition in the right column.

   _____ incontinence   a. Better rhythmic muscle contraction

   _____ peristalsis   b. Pus in the urine

   _____ defecation   c. Painful or difficult urination

   _____ flatulence   d. Bacteria in the urine

   _____ pyuria   e. Uncontrolled loss of urine or stool

   _____ bacteriuria   f. Evacuation of stool from the rectum

   _____ dysuria   g. Inability to completely empty the bladder during micturition

   _____ retention   h. Discharge of gas from the rectum

2. Which of the following body structures varies significantly between men and women?

   a. Urethra

   b. Ureter

   c. Bladder

   d. Sigmoid colon

3. Which of the following muscles allows adults to postpone urination?

   a. Detrusor

   b. Urogenital diaphragm

   c. Valves of Houston

   d. Depressor

4. Which of the following conditions, if left uncorrected, can lead to urinary retention?

   a. Benign prostatic hypertrophy

   b. Diabetes

   c. Multiple sclerosis

   d. Cystitis

5. Which of the following foods promotes constipation?

   a. Cheese

   b. Chocolate

   c. Celery

   d. Popcorn

6. Mrs. Gibbons, 78 years old, was admitted to the hospital from a skilled nursing facility (SNF) for chest pain to rule out myocardial infarction. She has been in the SNF for two days, increasingly becoming disoriented and anxious. In report you hear that Mrs. Gibbons is unable to hold her urine after she recognizes the urge to void and becomes incontinent on the way to the bathroom. Which of the following types of incontinence is Mrs. Gibbons experiencing?

   a. Functional incontinence

   b. Urge incontinence

   c. Stress incontinence

   d. Total incontinence

7. Mr. Keppler has been admitted today as a preoperative patient scheduled for surgery tomorrow. His urinalysis results come back from the lab showing a moderate amount of leukocytes in his urine. Is this a finding that you should report to the surgeon?

   ❏ Yes

   ❏ No

8. A helpful strategy to suggest to clients who are experiencing urinary incontinence is to limit fluid intake.

   ❏ True

   ❏ False

9. Clients receiving enteral feedings can experience diarrhea. Which of the following best explains the reason for this?

   a. Digestion is impaired.

   b. The feedings contain a high osmolality.

   c. The feedings damage the GI mucosa.

   d. Clients who require enteral feedings are experiencing a high catabolic state.

10. A client receiving narcotic analgesics and sedatives has the potential of becoming constipated.

❑ True

❑ False

11. During the assessment, your client informs you that she takes mineral oil every day to keep her bowels moving regularly. Which of the following nursing actions would you recommend?

a. Do nothing; mineral oil is a commonly used laxative.

b. Provide education; mineral oil can interfere with vitamin absorption.

c. Advise against taking mineral oil; there are less harmful laxatives on the market.

12. The penis of clients who use a condom catheter to manage urinary incontinence must be assessed regularly. What is the reason for this?

a. To check for lesions or rashes

b. To check for leakage

c. To check for twisting of the condom catheter

d. All of the above

13. Your client is experiencing constipation. Upon digital examination you find the stool is very dry and hard. Which of the following types of enema would be indicated for this patient?

a. Kayexalate

b. Oil retention

c. Carminitive

d. Antibiotic

14. How would you position a client when preparing to administer an enema?

a. Left side lying

b. Right side lying

c. Prone

d. Semi-Fowler's

15. Which of the following is most likely to be a temporary bowel diversion?

a. Double-barrel stoma

b. End stoma

c. Ileostomy

d. Sigmoid colostomy

16. When administering a large-volume enema, the maximum height of the solution should not exceed 12 inches.

    ❑ True

    ❑ False

17. Mr. Stevenson is four days post-op for a colon resection. While you are changing his colostomy bag, you notice the skin barrier has come loose. Upon removal of the skin barrier, you notice that his skin is beginning to ulcerate. Which of the following is the best course of action?

    a. Remeasure the stoma and place a smaller opening pouch over the stoma.

    b. Cleanse the skin around the stoma with antibacterial solution prior to application of the skin barrier.

    c. Contact the enterostomal therapist for a consultation.

    d. Report these assessment findings to the surgeon.

18. Which of the following is the correct procedure when administering a large enema?

    a. Insert the catheter tip into the anal canal 6 inches.

    b. Instruct the client to hold the enema for 20 minutes.

    c. Ensure the solution temperature is between 99° and 102°F.

    d. Continue the enema administration if the client states cramping is present.

19. During report you learn that Mr. Young has acquired a nosocomial *Clostridium difficile* infection. Which of the following symptoms would you expect to find during your assessment?

    a. Constipation

    b. Diarrhea

    c. Urge urinary incontinence

    d. Hematuria

20. As you interview your patient, she informs you that she takes Ditropan for her urge urinary incontinence problem. Which of the following interventions would *not* be included in her therapeutic regimen to manage this condition?

    a. Decreasing the intake of bladder irritants such as caffeine and high acid juices

    b. Adhering to a regular timed voiding schedule

    c. Increasing fluids rich in electrolytes

Answer Keys

Chapter 1

1. b
2. True
3. True
4. c
5. d
6. a
7. False
8. d, e, c, f, b, h, a, g
9. a
10. True
11. b, d, c, a
12. b
13. c
14. False
15. True
16. a
17. True
18. True
19. Yes
20. d

Chapter 2

1. c, e, b, f, d, a
2. b
3. b
4. developing nursing practice standards
5. b
6. True
7. d
8. a
9. d
10. b
11. False
12. a
13. True
14. b
15. c
16. 7, 4, 1, 5, 8, 3, 9, 6, 2
17. a
18. a
19. a
20. False

Chapter 3

1. d
2. b
3. False
4. True
5. c
6. d
7. True
8. d
9. True
10. no
11. b
12. a
13. b, c, d, c, a
14. True
15. c
16. True
17. d
18. d
19. False
20. a

Chapter 4

1. c
2. b
3. True
4. b
5. b, c, a
6. d
7. b
8. c
9. c
10. True
11. b
12. False
13. True
14. b
15. Yes
16. c
17. a
18. c
19. False
20. d

Chapter 5

1. b, c, a

2. Disagree

3. a

4. True

5. d

6. Habit, Fear of making mistakes, Use of meaningless routines and rituals

7. True

8. c, a, b, e, d

9. Subjective, Objective, Subjective, Objective, Subjective, Objective

10. d

11. c

12. True

13. b

14. b

15. c

16. False

17. d

18. True

19. b

20. True

Chapter 6

1. c

2. b

3. b

4. a

5. b, a, d, c

6. False

7. d

8. False

9. d

10. c

11. 6, 3, 2, 1, 5, 4

12. True

13. a

14. a

15. True

16. True

17. a

18. d

19. True

20. c

Chapter 7

1. a

2. False

3. a

4. False

5. b

6. b

7. Risk for Disuse Syndrome or Rape-Trauma Syndrome

8. False

9. c

10. 4, 6, 3, 7, 1, 2, 5

11. a

12. c

13. a

14. d

15. No

16. b

Chapter 8

1. True

2. a

3. d, c, b, a, e

4. 2, 1, 3

5. c

6. b

7. False

8. b

9. a

10. b

11. b

12. No

13. Yes

14. False

15. Yes

16. a

17. True

18. a

19. c

20. b

Chapter 9

1. a
2. a
3. d, a, e, c, b
4. d
5. a
6. a
7. b
8. c
9. a
10. True
11. c
12. b
13. True
14. d
15. True
16. c
17. d
18. a
19. True
20. Agree

Chapter 10

1. b, d, e
2. b
3. d
4. a
5. a
6. Disagree
7. c
8. d
9. d
10. True
11. b
12. False
13. b

Chapter 11

1. a, b, c, e

2. a

3. False

4. Social, Therapeutic, Social, Social, Therapeutic

5. Agree

6. a

7. b

8. True

9. b, a, d, c

10. b

11. presence

12. b

13. False

14. c, b, a

15. True

16. d

Chapter 12

1. b

2. b, a, e, d, c

3. b, c, a

4. d

5. True

6. d

7. a

8. No

9. b, d, c, a

10. False

11. e, c, f, b, d, a

12. c

13. Yes

14. a

15. No

16. d

17. d

18. True

19. c

20. False

21. No

22. c

23. No

24. a

25. Yes

Chapter 13

1. d
2. b
3. a
4. c
5. d
6. False
7. a, c, d, b
8. b
9. c
10. a
11. b
12. True
13. d
14. d
15. No
16. True
17. b
18. Yes
19. learning plateau
20. c

Chapter 14

1. b
2. b
3. b
4. a
5. c
6. Agree
7. a
8. b
9. 5, 3, 2, 1, 4
10. a
11. a
12. True
13. False
14. False
15. d
16. b
17. True
18. d
19. True
20. False

Chapter 15

1. a, f, d, e, b, c

2. a

3. b

4. Treating the client as a unique individual, Protecting privacy and confidentiality, Using touch and personal space in a therapeutic manner, Respecting cultural differences, Decreasing anxiety through stress management techniques

5. 2, 4, 3, 1

6. b, e, d, h, g, f, c, a

7. False

8. b

9. d

10. a

11. Yes

12. False

13. d

14. b

15. a

Chapter 16

1. a, g, e, f, d, b, c

2. True

3. communication

4. d, c, b, a

5. b

6. False

7. c

8. True

9. c

10. b

11. Agree

12. d, a, e, c, b

13. a

14. c

15. False

Chapter 17

1. b
2. False
3. a
4. a
5. d
6. b, e, d, c, a
7. False
8. bond
9. d
10. c
11. 6, 7, 2, 3, 1, 5, 4
12. a
13. False
14. d
15. b
16. b
17. b
18. d
19. a
20. b

Chapter 18

1. c
2. d
3. False
4. a
5. a
6. d, a, c, b
7. a
8. True
9. a
10. Yes
11. False
12. c
13. b
14. a
15. True
16. b, c, d, g, f, a, e
17. d
18. a
19. Decreased visual activity, Poor vision in dimly lit areas, Less foot and toe lift when walking, Altered center of gravity, Slower reflexes, Impaired muscle control, Orthostatic hypotension, Urinary frequency
20. b

Chapter 19

1. d, a, b, c
2. d
3. True
4. c
5. d
6. False
7. b
8. c
9. b
10. False
11. b
12. True
13. High self-esteem
14. a
15. a

Chapter 20

1. a, c, g, d, h, e, f, b
2. c
3. False
4. a
5. False
6. b
7. d
8. c
9. f, a, e, g, d, h, c, b
10. secondary gain
11. True
12. b
13. a
14. b
15. a
16. b, c, e, d, a
17. d
18. Yes
19. False
20. b

Chapter 21

1. g, f, a, b, e, d, c
2. False
3. a
4. a
5. b
6. b
7. True
8. b
9. a
10. b
11. d, e, c, b, a
12. True
13. a
14. a
15. True
16. b, a, c
17. c
18. False
19. Disagree
20. False

Chapter 22

1. b
2. No
3. d
4. d, e, g, b, f, a, c
5. True
6. False
7. b
8. a
9. d
10. True
11. Licensure examination, Continuing education, Certification
12. c
13. d, c, a, b
14. b
15. b
16. Yes
17. True
18. b
19. c
20. Find and use a mentor or preceptor, Form working relationships with colleagues, Establish a professional network, Consult with colleagues, Introduce others to contacts, Provide support to colleagues, Develop and use collaboration

Chapter 23

1. b

2. c, b, d, a, e

3. 2, 4, 1, 3

4. b

5. c

6. a

7. True

8. a

9. Yes

10. c

11. False

12. Failure to monitor client states, Medication errors, Falls, Use of restraints

13. True

14. b

15. Yes

16. True

17. No

18. a

19. b

20. b

Chapter 24

1. e, a, b, d, c

2. False

3. b

4. b, d, e, f, c, a

5. False

6. Informed consent, Refusal of treatment, Use of scarce resources, Impact of cost containment initiatives, Incompetent health care providers

7. True

8. d

9. Yes

10. True

11. d

12. b

13. a

14. No

15. d, a, b, c

16. a

17. False

18. a

19. Yes

20. a

Chapter 25

1. False
2. d, b, f, a, e, c
3. c
4. c
5. False
6. c
7. b
8. c
9. a
10. True
11. The nurse's customers are the patient, co-workers, and the organization where he/she works. The nurse is also accountable to families, visitors, and the community.
12. d
13. b
14. Current knowledge base, Effective interpersonal skills, Caring and compassion, Mutual decision making with clients, Individualized care
15. d
16. Audit
17. 3, 5, 1, 4, 2
18. a
19. Yes
20. True

Chapter 26

1. True
2. False
3. b
4. d
5. b
6. c
7. False
8. True
9. d
10. d
11. Yes
12. d, a, f, e, c, b
13. a
14. False
15. c
16. False
17. b
18. a
19. b
20. c

Chapter 27

1. False
2. c, a, f, d, e, g, b
3. c
4. b
5. False
6. a
7. a
8. a
9. a
10. a
11. True
12. b, d, a, f, c, g, e, h
13. b
14. c
15. True
16. a
17. g, h, f, e, d, c, j, b, i, a
18. False
19. a
20. d
21. b
22. d
23. d
24. c
25. cystocele

Chapter 28

1. True
2. False
3. b
4. Yes
5. No
6. False
7. c
8. a
9. True
10. False
11. a
12. a
13. d
14. True
15. c
16. Yes
17. a
18. Yes
19. c
20. c, d, g, f, e, h, b, i, a, j

Chapter 29

1. False
2. c
3. False
4. Yes
5. c, b, a, d
6. b
7. c
8. False
9. Yes
10. No
11. d
12. b
13. c
14. a
15. Right client, Right medication, Right dose, Right route, Right time
16. No
17. c
18. c
19. c
20. False
21. True
22. No
23. a
24. d
25. a
26. c

Chapter 30

1. a
2. d, e, c, b, a
3. True
4. c, a, d, b
5. False
6. False
7. c
8. Agree
9. a
10. b
11. a, c, b
12. c
13. False
14. embolus
15. c
16. a
17. d, a, e, c, b
18. True
19. d
20. a
21. False
22. a
23. b
24. b
25. d

Chapter 31

1. f, a, e, g, h, d, c, b

2. c, b, a, d, e

3. 3, 2, 4, 1

4. b

5. True

6. b

7. a

8. d

9. b

10. False

11. Yes

12. b

13. d

14. 10, 7, 9, 1, 3, 4, 8, 6, 5, 2

15. False

Chapter 32

1. c

2. a

3. d

4. crackles

5. b

6. b

7. True

8. True

9. b

10. d

11. a

12. atelectasis

13. c

14. Yes

15. d

Chapter 33

1. False
2. a
3. b
4. d
5. b
6. False
7. c
8. True
9. b
10. d
11. b, i, c, f, g, h, e, a, d
12. False
13. a
14. c
15. b, c, a
16. No
17. True
18. e, a, b, f, d, c
19. No
20. True

Chapter 34

1. b
2. c
3. b
4. a
5. d
6. c, d, g, f, e, b, a
7. True
8. d
9. a
10. c
11. d
12. b
13. True
14. c
15. 2 hours
16. c
17. False
18. b
19. c
20. c

Chapter 35

1. b
2. d, f, a, b, e, c
3. b
4. True
5. c
6. a
7. c
8. b
9. a
10. a
11. c
12. c
13. b
14. d
15. c
16. c
17. d
18. b
19. False
20. b

Chapter 36

1. c
2. False
3. d
4. c
5. b
6. a
7. a
8. True
9. d
10. c
11. No
12. True
13. a
14. b
15. c
16. False
17. b
18. a
19. b
20. d

Chapter 37

1. d, a, b, c
2. b
3. b
4. b
5. True
6. False
7. False
8. a
9. a
10. a
11. a
12. True
13. c
14. True
15. False
16. a
17. No
18. b
19. b
20. b
21. a
22. c
23. a
24. False
25. False
26. b
27. d
28. b
29. b
30. Yes

Chapter 38

1. a
2. d
3. d
4. a
5. False
6. e, h, a, g, f, b, c, d
7. a
8. a
9. b
10. c
11. True
12. True
13. 4, 2, 1, 3
14. True
15. False
16. True
17. False
18. b
19. b
20. c
21. a
22. No
23. a
24. False
25. d

Chapter 39

1. e, a, f, h, b, d, c, g
2. a
3. a
4. a
5. a
6. a
7. Yes
8. False
9. b
10. True
11. b
12. d
13. b
14. a
15. a
16. False
17. c
18. c
19. b
20. c